The Castle Connolly
Guide To

The ABCs of HMOs

How To Get The Best
From Managed Care

THE CASTLE CONNOLLY GUIDE TO

THE ABCs of HMOs

How To Get The Best

From Managed Care

The Castle Connolly Guide To
The ABCs of HMOs
How To Get The Best From Managed Care

For more information, please contact Castle Connolly Medical Ltd., 150 East 58th Street, New York, New York 10155, 212-980-8230. E-mail: CCMedical@aol.com. Web site: http://www.bestdocs.com

ISBN 1883769-74-4

Price: $11.95

Printed in the United States of America

Table of Contents

Appendices

Acknowledgements

Castle Connolly Medical Advisory Board

We are pleased to have associated with Castle Connolly Medical Ltd. a distinguished group of medical leaders who offer invaluable advice and wisdom in our efforts to assist consumers in obtaining the best health care.

Charles Bechert, M.D.
Director
The Sight Foundation
Fort Lauderdale, FL

Roger Bulger, M.D.
President
Association of Academic
Health Centers
Washington, DC

Harry J. Buncke, M.D.
Davies Medical Center
San Francisco, CA

Paul T. Calabresi, M.D.
Professor of Medicine and
  Medical Science
Chairman Emeritus
Department of Medicine
Brown University
Rhode Island Hospital
Providence, RI

Joseph Cimino, M.D.
Professor and Chairman
Community and
  Preventive Medicine
New York Medical College
Valhalla, NY

John C. Duffy, M.D.
Professor of Psychiatry
Department of Psychiatry
School of Medicine in
  New Orleans
Louisiana State University
  Medical Center
New Orleans, LA

J. Richard Gaintner, M.D.
Chief Executive Officer
Shands Health System
Gainsville, FL

Menard M. Gertler, M.D.,
  D. Sc.
Attending Physician
  Tisch Hospital
NYU Medical Center
New York, NY

Leo Hennikoff, M.D.
President and CEO
Rush Presbyterian-
  St.Luke's Medical Center
Chicago, IL

Yutaka Kikkawa, M.D.
Professor and Chairman
Department of Pathology
University of California
Irvine College of Medicine
Irvine, CA

Nicholas F. LaRusso, M.D.
Chairman
Division of Gastroenterology
Mayo Medical School
Clinic and Foundation
Rochester, MN

Benedict S. Maniscalco, M.D.
Chief Executive Officer
Access America Medical
  Care Inc.
Tampa, FL

David Paige, M.D.
Professor
Department of Maternal
  and Child Health
Johns Hopkins University
Baltimore, MD

Ronald Pion, M.D.
Chairman and CEO
Medical
  Telecommunicators Assoc.
Los Angeles, CA

James Sammons, M.D.
Haines City, FL

Leon G. Smith, M.D.
Director of Medicine and
Chief of Infectious Diseases
St. Michael's Medical
  Center
Newark, NJ

Ralph Snyderman, M.D.
Chancellor for Health
  Affairs
Duke University School of
  Medicine
Durham, NC

We would like to thank the physicians, health care leaders, and friends who took the time to review this manuscript and offer their thoughts and criticisms. We would particularly like to thank the following people for their hard work in the production of this book:

Editor: Sue Berkman

Assistant Editor: Fred Ramen

Consulting Editors: Dwight Langhum, Cathy Granata, Michael Wolf, Ph.D

Publications Coordinator: Adrienne Bonaparte

Cover and Interior Design and Production: Lissa Milea, Harper & Case, Ltd., NYC

Research Assistant: Connie Johnson

Foreword

Nothing brings you closer to reality than being a physician. For 25 years, as a practicing physician, editor, and commentator, I've grappled with HMO realities. Do HMOs provide good care? Do HMOs lower costs? At what human price? Are HMOs good for patients? Do HMOs improve quality? Do HMOs, as their name promises, maintain health? What are the real HMO trade-offs? As a physician I can vouch for the fact that this book intelligently and accurately responds to these questions.

When you consider health care marketplace realities, this book's timing is excellent. The market has spoken. Nationwide it is picking HMOs over traditional indemnity plans. Most big health care buyers — both in corporations and government — embrace market-driven HMOs to reduce costs. HMO growth has exploded since the Clinton plan imploded. As I write, 64 million Americans belong to HMOs. Another 101 million are enrolled in PPOs. By the year 2000, 200 million Americans will be members of these organizations.

The reality is that managed care is now the medical mainstream here in America. Nearly 85 percent of physicians now contract with HMOs. For doctors to practice, they must now accept HMOs as their economic lifeblood. Managed care is now rampantly replacing the old fee-for-service system. Why?

Because managed care controls premiums, lowers costs, and now satisfies most enrollees most of the time.

This, then, is a book of the here and now, not of the then and there. It is a practical, not a theoretical book. The book roots itself in managed care realities: It says plainly that the main reality for HMO enrollees is choice versus cost. If you want the old-style unlimited choice of doctors, hospitals, and benefits, you'll pay more for it. If you want lower premiums with less choice, you'll choose HMOs. And you'll receive care that compares favorably with fee-for-service care.

The book says plainly that HMOs are here to stay, that some are better than others, and that you'll have to do your homework and ask the right questions to pick the right one. It even gives you a useful form to calculate the best HMO based on the needs and preferences of your family, and a list of penetrating questions to ask.

It says plainly what the managed care alphabet soup — HMOs, PPOs, POSs, PHOs, EPOs, and PPMs — is all about. It doesn't bewail the managed care world's complexities. It confronts them, simplifies them, and tells you how to sort them out. To wit: The important thing to remember is that all these acronyms represent different organizational forms. They all take specific steps to control the use of resources and to control costs.

It says plainly what capitation means and portends: The practice of capitation, now common in HMO agreements with doctors, is at the heart of managed care philosophically, financially and operationally. It is a fundamental principle for putting the provider of care at risk for the cost of the care provided. The logic behind capitation makes sense. If doctors' decisions are behind 85 percent of health care expenditures, give them financial responsibility as well as medical responsibility.

It says plainly why most doctors don't like HMOs. In many physicians' eyes, HMOs negatively impact their independence, interfere with patient relationships, lower quality, discount fees, monitor their activities, challenge their clinical judgment, and judge their patients' satisfaction. Doctors' negative opinions have not slowed HMOs' momentum. Most doctors now have contracts with HMOs because they have little choice. HMOs control 50 to 60 percent of many major metropolitan markets. As a physician, you can dislike HMOs, but you can't ignore them or hide from them.

It says plainly that HMOs have pitfalls for some Americans: Older Americans may have to leave their longtime doctors, those with mental disease may be restricted to a number of paid visits, those who are dying may be denied heroic or experimental treatment, those who desire certain care — cosmetic surgery, sex change operations or chiropractic care — may be excluded from that care, and those who seek care in an emergency room or locations outside the HMO's sphere of coverage may find that payment will not be forthcoming from the HMO.

But on the whole, it says plainly that the American public and the other participants in the system — buyers, hospitals, physicians, other providers, and suppliers — have recognized that HMOs and other forms of managed care are now the dominant force in health care and have brought about reform as radical as any proposed by the government. It is, as the authors tell us, the new reality and one to which doctors, hospitals — and especially consumers — must adapt.

In short, this is an honest book, plainly told, and anyone who contemplates joining or switching HMOs, or who is now in an HMO, will benefit from it.

Richard L. Reece, M.D.
Editor, *Physician Practice Options*
Chairman, National Association of
Integrated Health Organizations

Part One

1

AN OVERVIEW

Highlights

Much of what we read and hear about managed care and HMOs is negative. Yet, for most Americans managed care is the new reality. This chapter describes the media and political response to managed care, and how ordinary citizens are struggling to deal with this new way of delivering health care. The goals of the book are spelled out, as well as the need and urgency for consumers to become better informed.

QUESTIONS ANSWERED IN THIS CHAPTER INCLUDE:

Why should I spend time reading this book?

What will I get out of it?

Who should I believe, the critics or supporters of managed care?

Are all the negative things I read and hear about managed care true?

The ABCs of HMOs

WHAT'S IN IT FOR YOU?

In a crowded elevator in New York City, two men discuss their work day:
"A big envelope from our new health plan was waiting on everybody's desk. Nobody knew that it was coming and everybody has a lot of questions about this plan since it seemed to offer so many more benefits than the medical plan we used to have."

In a day care center in Minnesota two mothers watch their toddlers play:
"My husband's employer signed up with an HMO plan that doesn't list very many pediatricians and I'm concerned because ours isn't on the list."

In a restaurant in Denver a husband and wife wait for their meal:
"I read in a newspaper the other day about a woman who was diagnosed with breast cancer and her doctor recommended a new treatment, but her health plan refused to authorize payment because they considered it experimental. Could that happen to me in our plan?"

All across the country, people in elevators, restaurants, day care centers, people like you — members of your family, your friends, and neighbors — are discussing the pros and cons of, and looking for definitive answers to, the mysteries of HMOs (Health Maintenance Organizations), and an understanding of that ambiguous term "managed care," the new reality of health care in the United States.

While their search for answers goes on, and while employers and the government encourage and even mandate health insurance through managed care companies, they read headlines like the following:

"The Lethal Side Effects of Managed Care"
- Business Week

"Torture by HMO"
- New York Times

"Managed Care's Seamy Side"
- Modern Healthcare

"The HMO Hazard"
- Washington Post

"Medicine Aches with HMO Fever"
- Chicago Tribune

"Beware Your HMO"
- Newsweek

"Docs Say HMOs Add Insult to Injury"
- Boston Globe

No wonder that a survey by the National Coalition on Health Care and International Communications Research found that 79 percent of Americans polled felt "there is something wrong with our health care system" and fewer than half the people surveyed felt they have "confidence in the health care system to take care of me"; or that a *Chicago Sun-Times*/KPMG Peat Marwick health benefits survey reported that 66 percent of its respondents said they felt that managed care's main goal is to save money for corporations.

Perhaps the use of the word "system" to describe the way we deliver health care in this nation is itself inaccurate. To most consumers, health care in the United States is not a system, but a confusing mess of organizations, acronyms, and governmental agencies all claiming a piece of the patient. Running throughout is a deep concern and a lack of trust on the part of consumers and patients. However, and most central to this book, whatever our "system," or lack of one, managed care is an important — and growing — part of it.

Are the headlines accurate? Should people fear managed care, or is managed care a new way of delivering health care that can provide quality care at lower costs? Who is telling the truth — managed care's critics, or its supporters?

Right now there are few final answers. Hundreds of HMOs have sprung up across the country in the last ten years. Each one is different from the others, or so it seems. Some are very good; some are not. Worse, there is no central source of information on HMOs and no across-the-board method of rating them, so it is difficult to make the right choice — if you have a choice! But all that is changing.

To complicate matters, the process of choosing a health plan is not a one-time event; it occurs every year, and even more often for some people. You may want to change your health plan; your employer may offer different plans from one year to the next; you may change jobs; or your company may merge and you may have

A TOWERS PERRIN SURVEY SHOWED THAT FOR SUPPORT IN MAKING HEALTH CARE DECISIONS, ADVERTISING (2 PERCENT), THE MEDIA (6 PERCENT) AND GOVERNMENT (8 PERCENT) WERE *LEAST* TRUSTED BY AMERICANS WHILE DOCTORS WERE MOST TRUSTED (62 PERCENT). HMOS SCORED 14 PERCENT.

to change plans. Whatever the reason, choosing a health plan is a major decision point in your life or the life of your family. Even if you know that it's not a permanent decision, the choice should be made as though it were a matter of life and death. It very well could be.

Books and articles about managed care seem to come from one of two perspectives. The first point of view is that of those who believe managed care, especially HMOs, is the answer to all the problems of our health care system, while the second take is from those who believe managed care organizations are the scourge of humanity, denying people care and making fortunes for their executives and stockholders.

This book approaches the topic with neither bias. Just as there are good doctors and poor doctors, there are good managed care plans and poor managed care plans. This book has three goals: (1) *to help you understand managed care and how it functions*; (2) *to help you distinguish between good and poor managed care plans, so that you can make the best choices*; and (3) *to help you get the best care possible once you are in a managed care plan*. [Note: Throughout this book we will use a number of terms interchangeably to describe managed care: Health Maintenance Organization (HMO); health plan; managed health plan; and managed care organization (MCO). Technically, an HMO is but one form of managed care; a description of the other forms follows later in chapter 4.]

Whether it is for better or for worse our health care system has changed dramatically in the last ten years or so. While some of the changes may be good — such as bringing costs under control — one of the significant negatives is the loss of trust most people have in our health care system and even in their own health care providers: doctors, hospitals and insurers. The result of this change is that individuals and families need to prepare themselves — to be empowered — to deal with the new system we face. As John Rother, American Association of Retired Persons (AARP) Director of Legislation and Public Policy wrote in *Modern Maturity*, "Consumers will be challenged to be better informed and more vigilant as health care becomes more bottom line oriented. More coordinated approaches to the health of our communities show great promise not only for improving the health-care system but also for making it more cost-effective. But the price of this progress is the necessity for consumers and patients to be more informed, more a part of medical decisions, and more sensitive to the need to use medical services appropriately."

People can no longer be passive patients. They must assume greater responsibility for their health care. They must be assertive consumers to be certain they, and their families, get the best care possible. This book will guide you in that process.

To help achieve these goals we have made this book not only useful, but as user-friendly as possible. The chapters are arranged in a logical progression, starting from the very moment you are faced with making a choice of

A KAISER FAMILY FOUNDATION STUDY SHOWED THAT OVER HALF WOULD SELECT A HEALTH PLAN RECOMMENDED BY FAMILY AND FRIENDS OVER ONE RATED MUCH HIGHER BY INDEPENDENT ORGANIZATIONS THAT RATE HEALTH PLANS.

OVER HALF, 55
PERCENT, OF
THOSE PEOPLE
SURVEYED BY
LOUIS HARRIS
AND ASSOCIATES
AND TOWERS
PERRIN, HAD
NEVER HEARD OF
THE TERM *MAN-
AGED CARE.*
ALMOST A
THIRD, 31 PER-
CENT, SAID THEY
NEVER HEARD OF
THE TERM HMO.

an HMO or managed care plan through to the many choices you may need to make once you are enrolled. We have provided personal stories related to us by family, friends, friends of friends, and associates about their encounters with HMOs and other managed care plans in order to give examples of how some of the principles and policies of managed care work in real life, not simply in theory.

Furthermore, we are keenly aware that when it comes to media reporting of managed care issues, the headlines are full of controversies, often extrapolated from a single case based on its sensationalism, without any real resolutions. Yet such individual examples are and should be troubling. Although they may distort the true image of managed care and are isolated events, they can also be accurate reflections of major failings.

Clearly, one thing they have achieved is to stimulate serious consumer and political backlash against managed care in communities. In many of the chapters that follow, we have addressed the most visible and controversial issues in a balanced way that we believe will educate and enlighten you, and help you deal effectively with the issues if you confront them. Finally, we have provided recommendations of additional sources of information to use in your ongoing search for the best health care for yourself and your family.

•Issues and Controversy•

"Gag Clauses"

"Gag clauses" is the term applied to an issue that stirred up a great deal of controversy in early 1996. Brought to a head by a Boston doctor who claimed he was terminated by an HMO because he criticized their policy of restricting what doctors could tell patients about treatment alternatives, the issue attracted national attention when it was found that many HMOs had similar clauses in their agreements.

This produced a rash of laws and regulations on the part of various state legislatures to prohibit such clauses. Many of the HMOs that had similar clauses dropped them. The federal government also took action and issued a strong order to HMOs, restricting such clauses in contracts for service to Medicare patients.

This whole issue has been a public relations nightmare for managed care organizations. They were put in the position of appearing to restrict a doctor's communications with patients. The essence of the issue concerned doctors discussing with patients the best possible treatment options, even if they were not covered by the plan. The public and political leaders were properly outraged by the notion that such conversations may have been prohibited, and the managed care industry reacted to the firestorm by adopting a statement opposing such clauses. The American Association of Health Plans adopted its "Putting Patients First" initiative (Appendix E) in December of 1996, which not only proposed improved communication with physicians and patients, but also dealt with issues such as precertification, physician compensation and formularies.

At the same time, the issue is not quite as simple as the HMO critics made it seem. While very few HMOs, if any, terminated doctors who were critical of their policies, many HMOs had various types of clauses in their contracts with doctors that they felt were justified. For example, HMOs typically have clauses restricting doctors from talking about other HMOs with patients. Their concern is a basic one: If a doctor is going to leave one HMO to join another, they don't want that doctor recruiting his or her patients for the new HMO.

HMO contracts also frequently have sections that prohibit doctors from making derogatory remarks about the plan that would undermine a patient's confidence in the quality of care. Some of these stipulations do protect patients and some may be intended to protect the HMO from criticism.

Ask any HMO you are considering, or if you are in an HMO ask your doctor, if it has such a clause. These days most HMOs have backed off such limitations if they had them. If your HMO does have such a clause, ask your doctor if it will limit your care options or his or her ability to discuss options with you. You have to be confident that nothing will restrict your receiving necessary care.

Notes & Phone Numbers

Highlights

For most Americans, the world of health care insurance has changed drastically in recent years. From indemnity insurance to managed care, from trusting health providers to questioning who is really watching out for patients, things are radically different.

QUESTIONS ANSWERED IN THIS CHAPTER INCLUDE:

What is the difference between managed care and indemnity insurance coverage?

How does managed care pay doctors and hospitals?

How has the fee-for-service system affected health costs?

Where, how, and when did HMOs begin and grow?

Why is it critical for consumers to understand choices in managed care?

Managed Care

A NEW WAY OF DELIVERING HEALTH CARE

At one time health care costs for most Americans were covered by a form of insurance known as indemnity health insurance. Usually, such insurance was offered by an employer as part of a salary package; people came to understand that medical "benefits" were an important part of their compensation. The term indemnity comes from indemnify, which means to protect against loss. As applied to health insurance, indemnity protects against the financial loss that could result from large bills incurred during an illness or injury. You may remember what it was like: You went to the doctor and/or a hospital, paid the bill, and then sought reimbursement from the insurance company, or submitted the bill to the insurance company to pay.

Hospitals were paid in a number of different ways, but typically it was on a per diem (daily rate) basis. That meant whatever your reason for being hospitalized, the hospital would receive the same set amount per day from insurers. For the most part indemnity insurance covered about 80 percent of a hospital stay.

Doctors were paid on a "fee-for-service" basis. That is, they were paid fees based on the services they performed. Usually an insurance company would pay on what was termed a "usual and customary" fee schedule, meaning the fee typically charged for that service in that community. Frequently, especially in large metropolitan cities such as New York, Chicago, San Francisco, and Dallas, doctor's fees exceeded the insurance company's fee schedule. Consequently, patients often were left to pay the remaining sum of money to the doctor after the insurance company had come up with their top dollar. Such out-of-pocket expenses were often a burden for patients.

The indemnity, fee-for-service arrangement had larger problems. Most significantly, the whole system of payments incorporated built-in incentives to doctors and other health care providers to do more and to charge more. The more services a doctor performed, the more he or she would be paid, whether or not those services were required or necessary. The more a hospital charged, the higher its daily rate would become and the more it would be reimbursed. Since most hospitalizations, but very little outpatient care, were covered by insurance, it was to everyone's advantage — doctors, hospitals, and patients — to hospitalize patients for care rather than treating them in less expensive outpatient settings. In fact, our health care system was centered around hospitals, and keeping them at full occupancy was a major goal.

The entire health care financing system was geared to more use and higher fees. Health care costs escalated to the point that health care was consuming about 14 percent of the nation's gross national product (GNP) in 1996.

Critics of the system also complained that indemnity insurance was geared towards illness, not wellness; the only time indemnity insurers paid was when a person was sick. It was extremely rare, and still is, for any indemnity insurance company to pay a doctor for preventive care. Since there was no system for organizing and delivering preventive care — it all depended on how interested you and your doctor were in it — and no system for paying doctors to deliver that kind of care, there was little preventive care delivered. A doctor might have reminded you to stop smoking, lose weight, etc., but rarely would a doctor have the time or interest to organize and mount an effective program to accomplish these goals. Prevention was simply not an important issue in health care.

Indemnity insurance and the conditions described still exist, but only for a minority of people who can afford a system with few restraints.

Cost Versus Choice

An alternative form of health care delivery and insurance existed in the form of HMOs, but it was relatively unknown to consumers in most of the country until the last 15 years. HMOs were the first and best known form of what we term broadly as "managed care." Today's HMOs trace their roots to 1945 and the establishment of the Kaiser Foundation Health Plan. Although there are other and earlier examples of health programs with some elements of HMOs, it was really the Kaiser Plan that began the "modern era" of HMOs. The growth of HMOs was stimulated by a federal law, known as the

HEALTH INSURANCE, ACCORDING TO AN EMPLOYEE BENEFITS INSTITUTE SURVEY, IS THE BENEFIT CONSIDERED MOST IMPORTANT BY ADULTS WHEN CONSIDERING A JOB.

Health Maintenance Organization Act, passed in 1973 in response to rapidly rising health care costs. This act made HMOs part of federal health policy. Basically, it allowed the federal government to mandate that employers with 25 or more employees had to offer federally qualified HMOs as a health insurance option unless they were self-insured. To be federally qualified under the law, an HMO had to provide an extensive set of benefits and coverages, demonstrate financial stability and ensure provider (hospital and doctor) participation.

HMOs are the best-known form of managed care, combining insurance and medical services. In other words, an HMO is a system of organizing, delivering, and financing health care. When an HMO accepts a fixed fee for providing all of a person's care, including hospitalization, it also accepts a risk. The HMO bets that the combined payment from all members will be greater than the total cost of providing the care needed by all members. Because of this risk, the HMO must manage the care delivered to be certain the costs do not exceed the revenues. It is really an insurance company that doesn't just pay bills, but organizes and delivers health care.

The greatest stimulant to the tremendous growth of managed care in the last decade has not been the federal government, but private employers. Concerned about the impact of rapidly rising costs of health care provided as a benefit to employees and their families, employers looked to managed care to control those costs and to make them more predictable. Now the government has given managed care a significant edge by viewing it as a way to control the rapidly rising costs of Medicare and Medicaid. As a result, enrollments in HMOs and other kinds of managed care plans have surged and managed care has delivered the cost control it promised. The rapid increase in health costs experienced during the 1980s has slowed and health costs are now more predictable and increasing less rapidly.

The issue of predictability in costs is at the very heart of managed care plans. When first created, they were known as "pre-paid" health plans because providers were paid even before care was given. Unlike indemnity health insurance plans (the type many of us were used to), where the insurance company pays the bill only after care is delivered, HMOs and other pre-paid plans receive payment on a monthly basis regardless of how much care is delivered.

SEVENTY THREE PERCENT OF U.S. WORKERS ARE IN SOME FORM OF MANAGED CARE.

Under indemnity insurance, rates charged to employers can increase substantially based on "experience" (the use and costs of care). If the prior year's bills were more than the insurance company had projected, the insurance bill could rise dramatically. If they were lower, the insurance company made a larger profit. However, the direction of employer's bills during this period went one way — up. If the employer was self-insured, and paid employees' health care bills directly, that increase could hit the company's budget that same year.

Managed Care Is Here to Stay

Indemnity insurance will be a fact of American life for many years to come, available to those who can afford it and want unlimited choice of doctors and hospitals without restraint. But, as the following chart illustrates, managed care has grown tremendously in the last ten years and is projected to grow even more in coming years.

Historical and Projected HMO Enrollment, 1980–2000

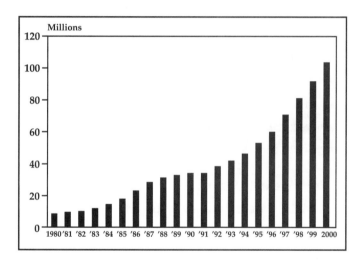

Nationally, over 150 million people are enrolled in some form of managed care. Over 70 percent of insured employees have some limits on their choice of doctors because of a managed care element of their health insurance. Enrollment in the nation's 660 plus HMOs grew by about 10 percent in 1996, according to

Interstudy, the not-for-profit group that tracks managed care. Approximately 65 million people in the U.S. belong to HMOs, a sixfold increase from the 10.2 million in 1982. Another 90 million belong to PPOs. HMOs in this country are signing up new members at the rate of 14,000 a day! (The most rapid growth has been in the Independent Practice Association (IPA) model, which now accounts for about 53 percent of all HMOs and 45 percent of all HMO enrollment. Insurance companies now own more than one-third of all HMOs).

HMOs and other forms of managed care are here and here to stay, at least for the foreseeable future. Doctors and hospitals are coming to terms with the new health care environment and patients must learn to do so as well.

Chance or Choice: It's Up to You

One of the prevailing misconceptions about managed care is that participants in these plans completely lose their freedom of choice. To some extent this is true when choosing a health plan because many employers — over half, in fact — contract with only a single health plan, which means that all employees must participate in that plan or pay for health care on their own. But many other employers (especially large ones) offer their workers some choice of health care plans. Over 65 percent of "jumbo" employers (over 5,000 employees) offer at least three health plans to their employees, according to a KPMG, Peat Marwick study. A study published in the prestigious journal *Health Affairs* reported that 62 percent of workers have a choice of at least two health plans. While it is true that some 40 percent of those who join HMOs and other managed care plans do have to leave their current doctor in order to sign on with a participating doctor, the choices of primary care doctors within a plan are usually numerous and, in some cases, even overwhelming. This may be less true of the choice of other kinds of specialists and of hospitals because managed care organizations are designed to limit these selections; however, some choice is usually offered, even if it is limited in some way. Since choice is critically important to most of us, one purpose of this book is to help you make informed choices every step of the way and to help you broaden your choices whenever possible by understanding how managed care operates.

FOUR TIMES AS MANY EMPLOYEES ARE ENROLLED IN MANAGED CARE HEALTH PLANS THAN IN INDEMNITY HEALTH PLANS.

•Issues and Controversy•

Cherry Picking

From the earliest days of HMOs, critics have contended that the positive results of lower cost and good health status claimed by HMOs were a result of their selecting younger, healthier members — "cherry picking" — and avoiding older, less healthy populations.

Actually the issue of selective underwriting on the part of insurance companies has always been with us. Some insurance companies always have attempted to enroll healthier people. This is true under indemnity insurance as well as under managed care. An insurance company could hardly offer competitive rates if it enrolled only sick patients. In fact, this point has been made dramatically by the financial struggles of many Blue Cross/Blue Shield organizations, who are often required by state regulators to accept anyone who applies for insurance. As they accepted these high-risk members in greater numbers than many other insurers, their rates climbed and their prices became less competitive, thus drawing off more of those who were healthy and could afford to leave for other insurers. The "Blues" were left with growing populations of those who could not get insurance elsewhere, and consequently, ever increasing rates. This vicious cycle led to the bankruptcy of some "Blues."

A continuing concern regarding managed care is the ability (or desire) of some health plans to adequately serve chronically ill patients. Whether it is by making referrals to specialists more difficult, discouraging enrollment of chronically ill patients, or having too few specialists to serve that population, this area has become a primary focus of concern for these patients, their families, and the "watchdogs" of managed care.

Insurance companies do not go out of their way to sell insurance to sick people under any system. Recently, for example, managed care organizations have been criticized for enrolling only the healthier segment of the Medicare population. Managed care supporters argue that is not the case. It is up to state or federal regulators to make certain there is a way for those who cannot obtain insurance in a competitive market to obtain it through other means and that the cost of this is shared fairly. Whether that solution requires private insurers to accept a proportion of those people, or the creation of a new program, the concept of insurance rests on the principle that we all share the risks and costs to protect any of us from catastrophic expenses.

This concept does not work well in a highly competitive market unless the government sets some rules. While we want competition to thrive, and realize it will bring lower costs and higher quality, we have to ensure adequate access to health care for all our citizens.

One thing is true about HMOs in this regard. They tend to attract younger people who are healthier. Because younger people believe they are not going to need much health care, they frequently seek the lowest cost, most hassle-free option and, in most cases, that's an HMO. However, with the tremendous growth of managed care, which is now covering broader segments of the population, those demographics are changing.

Part Two

HOW TO CHOOSE THE BEST MANAGED CARE PLAN

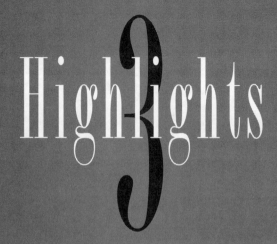

Highlights

Quality is the single most important issue to many people, but few people know how to measure the quality of their health plan. The basic factors to be considered in choosing a plan are model, coverages, cost and quality.

QUESTIONS ANSWERED IN THIS CHAPTER INCLUDE:

What are group, staff, and IPA models?

How can I plan coverages to best meet my family's needs?

How can I assess the real cost of an HMO plan?

Where can I obtain basic information on a health plan?

Making 3 Choices

FOUR STEPS
TO THE BEST HMO

To many people, selecting an HMO or other managed care plan is simple. If their doctor is in the network, it's a good plan; if their doctor is not in the network, it's not a good plan. In reality, while having a doctor you trust and respect is critically important, it should not be the only consideration. When selecting among HMOs there are a number of important factors to consider. The following pages describe these factors, where to find the information you need, how to assess that information, and how to use it to make the best choices.

This chapter provides a brief overview. Successive chapters will review each of the important characteristics of managed care you should consider in greater depth when making your choices.

The four basic factors you should assess when selecting an HMO are: model, coverages, cost, and quality. Each of these factors is divided into a number of subparts for your consideration. The information to answer all questions posed should be available from the HMOs you are considering. Some of the information may be obtained from accrediting bodies or from state agencies. Your employer also may be a good source of information on the plans it is offering. Typically the opportunity to choose a health insurance plan offered by your employer occurs only once or twice a year during what is called "open enrollment." It is usually at this time that employers and HMOs will distribute written material and hold informational meetings. Open enrollment is usually in September or October, although June is also a popular month.

Model

One very important consideration is the model or type of HMO. Is it a model in which all of the doctors are in one central location (staff or group model), or is it an Independent Practice Association (IPA), with the doctors providing most care in their own private offices? In either case, is it a Point of Service (POS) plan which allows you the option to seek care outside of the network? Consider which you prefer, and how comfortable you feel with each.

Coverages

HMOs offer different plans and each differs greatly in its coverages. Also, coverages are usually related to cost. If you pay more, you generally get more, but the relationship is not exact. In assessing different coverages, judge them as they relate to your needs and those of your family. A broad coverage you don't need is not of great value to you, but skimpy coverage for a service you may need often is a significant drawback. Despite the common impression that HMOs cover every health need, many managed health plans do not necessarily cover all services. There are some not covered at all, called exclusions. There are also some services that will be limited or "capped." You should examine the coverages offered by plans you are considering carefully.

Chapter 5 outlines the types of coverages offered by HMOs and describes what high-end (extensive) or low-end (less extensive) coverage might be for each benefit or service. These are just examples, and plans may offer somewhat different forms of coverages, but chapter 5 gives you a guide for assessing each coverage in any plan you are considering.

Cost

Cost is related to coverages. In judging whether or not a plan is a good buy you must first assess the coverages as they relate to your needs. Also, not only is it important to judge overall cost because it is possible that you and your employer are sharing this expense, but it is also important to judge **your** out-of-pocket expenses based on how you use health care. For example, if you're young and healthy and rarely see a doctor except for annual exams, a high deductible or copay provision may not be a problem. On the other hand, if you have a chronic condition and need to visit a doctor regularly, a high copay for each visit may be a consideration. In the same vein, if you are on regular, expensive medications, the drug plan is of great importance. Consider carefully and honestly how you and your family use health care resources.

IN AN AMA POLL, 77 PERCENT OF THE PEOPLE SURVEYED SAID THEY WOULD PAY MORE FOR HEALTH CARE IF THEY COULD PICK THEIR OWN PHYSICIANS.

Quality

Quality is a complex factor. We have divided it into four parts for consideration: accreditation, provider network, service, and outcomes. Each of these is examined separately. Quality is the most difficult characteristic to assess, but there are ways to do so that are undeniably worth the time and effort.

Getting the Facts on Health Plans

Health plans are usually very willing to provide prospective members with literature describing their mode of operation. When evaluating this literature, try to answer the questions on the following pages. If you cannot, call the organization's office. When you have answered all of them, sit down with your family and discuss the options. The choice you make among HMOs, other managed care plans, or fee-for service care should be based upon your preferences and needs. If you are not clear on the answers to the questions outlined in this book, call or visit the HMO. If there is a central location where all care is provided, a visit is a good idea in any case, so you can assess the physical plant, cleanliness of the facilities, and attitude and courtesy of the staff. In the case of an IPA model, visit the doctor you want as your primary care doctor. Get a sense of his or her office, staff and location if possible.

Ask questions and get assessments about the plan, including opinions and ideas from the people in the organization as well as from as many people as you know who are enrolled in the plan. Research has shown that most people give ratings of family and friends a great deal of weight in making choices of health plans and providers.

HMOs, like other insurers, typically offer a variety of plans. Usually the offerings are determined by your employer who, in most cases, is the major payer. Remember, most employers permit changes in health plans only during a selected period each year.

The information that follows focuses on a number of important factors you will want to assess when choosing an HMO. We previously have raised the question of the model or form of managed care, and that is an issue you and your family should think through. The additional characteristics you should consider are related to coverages, cost, and quality. Finding a balance of all these characteristics is the key to the best choice of an HMO.

A SURVEY BY THE COMMON-WEALTH FUND FOUND THAT YOUNGER WOMEN WERE MORE LIKELY TO JOIN HMOS THAN OLDER WOMEN.

•Issues and Controversy•

Lifetime Caps

An issue that has attracted little press attention to date, but is a very critical one to all families, is that of yearly or lifetime expenditure caps. Simply translated, this means a limit on the dollar amount an insurance company will be responsible for during a year or during the lifetime of a policy. It applies in both indemnity and managed care situations. While it affects very few people, it can have a devastating impact on those it does affect.

Some insurance policies have limits of $250,000 a year or a million dollars in a lifetime. While these seem to be huge amounts, they can disappear rapidly in today's expensive hi-tech medical environment, where life saving miracles occur daily, but often at great expense. This issue was vividly brought to the attention of our nation by the tragic case of Christopher Reeve, the film star best known for his work as Superman, who became a quadriplegic after a fall from a horse. Despite his wealth, he found himself impoverished in less than two years as the result of his expensive care and the limits of his insurance.

Families should seek insurance plans, managed care or indemnity, without caps or limits.

Notes & Phone Numbers

Highlights

4

Acronyms and new terms confuse many consumers who then "give up" before attempting to understand managed care. This chapter defines the most common terms and explains how the organizations they describe affect consumers.

QUESTIONS ANSWERED IN THIS CHAPTER INCLUDE:

What is an MCO?

How do group, staff and IPA models differ?

What is a PPO, EPO, POS, PHO?

What are Physician Practice Management (PPM) Companies?

Models

MAKING SENSE OF
THE ALPHABET SOUP

It is confusing enough to try to understand medical terms, doctor's recommendations, names of drugs and all the rest of the vocabulary that directly relates to your state of sickness or health. Now there is a new language to learn — one comprised entirely of acronyms that stand for the various types of managed care organizations that deliver health care. But make no mistake, these cryptic names also relate directly to your state of sickness and health. Understanding what each of these managed care organizations is and how it functions will help you understand how to get the best care whether you're in an **HMO**, **PPO**, **PSO** or some other kind of plan.

The important thing to remember is that while all these acronyms represent different organizational forms, they share one common theme: They all take specific steps to control the use of health care resources (doctors, hospitals, tests) and to control costs; this is an important part of the definition of "managing care." All of these organizations fall under the umbrella heading of managed care organization (MCO). While most managed care organizations are concerned about quality, this concern extends only to the point that quality can be achieved along with cost control. Sometimes managed care organizations are accused of managing costs, not care!

In reality, the individual terms as well as the way they fit into the whole managed care picture are not so confusing at all, if you approach them one step at a time.

Health Maintenance Organization (HMO)

HMOs are the first and best known form of managed care. HMOs are usually what people think of as managed care and, in fact, HMO is the term that will appear most frequently in these pages because it is the most relevant form of MCO for most people. HMOs combine the insurance function and the provision of care. As a result, HMOs assume a financial risk. The risk is that the cost of care for the covered period (a year, for example) will not exceed the amount of the insurance premium paid by you or your employer. This is called "assuming risk."

HMOs, therefore, are motivated to control the cost of your care (so as not to exceed the premium) and to help you stay healthy and not use expensive resources (like a hospital) too frequently. They do this by "managing care."

Of course, like those of all insurers, the HMOs' premiums and cost projections are based on large populations, not individuals. This is a good place to point out the difference between managed health plans and indemnity style health insurance.

Under indemnity plans *you* choose your providers (doctors and hospitals) and the insurers pay the bills *after* they are submitted and deemed appropriate. You also pay whatever deductibles and copays are required. You also may have to pay the difference between what the insurer pays the doctor or hospital and the total amount of the bill — sometimes not an insubstantial amount.

Under managed care your costs are fixed, although there may be modest deductibles (rarely) and copays (usually). But in managed care, the insurer — an HMO, for example — selects the providers you can choose from, negotiates an amount your provider will receive for your care, and pays the bills *directly* instead of reimbursing you after you have paid them.

In exchange for generally lower costs and less paper work — and usually broader coverages — you trade off complete freedom of choice of providers and accept management of your care under the direction of the HMO.

HMOs may be organized in a number of different forms, or models:

Staff Model – The physicians are employees of the HMO and practice in one or more central locations where diagnostic and other facilities also may be located.

Group Model – The physicians are organized into one or more large medical groups and practice in one or more

A SURVEY BY THE CHICAGO BUSINESS GROUP ON HEALTH DEMONSTRATED THAT 84 PERCENT OF THOSE SURVEYED WERE SATISFIED WITH THEIR MANAGED CARE HEALTH PLAN.

central locations where diagnostic and other facilities may also be located. Group and staff model HMOs were the earliest models and gave rise to the impression that HMO members had to go to a "clinic" to receive care. Although largely an inaccurate perception, it did slow the growth of HMOs for many years. To consumers these models are virtually indistinguishable.

IPA – The Independent Practice Association model contracts with individual or groups of physicians to provide care to patients in the physicians' private offices. As such, the physician remains an independent contractor. This is now the most popular HMO model.

Network Model – The network model HMO engages multiple groups of physicians to provide care to patients. This model simply expands the group form into multiple locations.

Mixed Model – A mixed model HMO is any combination of the above.

Preferred Provider Organization (PPO)

This is another popular form of managed care. In fact, more people are enrolled in PPOs than in HMOs. A PPO is a group of providers — doctors, hospitals, or both — that provides care at a discounted rate. In turn, the covered population pays less if they receive care from the PPO, but pays more if they go outside the PPO network.

Exclusive Provider Organization (EPO)

This organization is similar to a PPO except that the insured population *must* receive all of its care from the EPO participating providers. If a member goes outside of the EPO network providers they are not covered and must pay the bills themselves.

The HMO and PPO are the principal forms of managed care. However, there are other acronyms you may see or hear in this rapidly changing health care environment which are clarified below.

Point of Service Plan (POS)

In this type of health plan offered by many HMOs, members may go outside of the HMO network to choose any provider they want. POS plans are among the most popular and fastest growing type of health plan because of their flexibility; however, when members exercise this choice they pay a larger portion of the costs. For example, instead of the HMO paying the entire bill, the HMO may only pay 70 percent and the member pays the balance.

THE AMERICAN ASSOCIATION OF HEALTH PLANS AND ERNST AND YOUNG REPORTED THAT 74 PERCENT OF HEALTH PLANS OFFERED A POINT OF SERVICE (POS) OPTION.

The Physician-Hospital Organization (PHO)

Doctors and hospitals may come together to function as a managed care plan, or may negotiate with managed care plans to provide services. In many cases they form a formal legal entity labeled a **Physician-Hospital Organization** (PHO). These organizations are created primarily by hospitals and their medical staffs to give them a stronger, united negotiating position with managed care organizations, which usually demand deep discounts from doctors and hospitals. Another term used is **Provider Service Organization** (PSO) which (in many cases) involves only doctors and not hospitals.

In either case, the number of PHOs and PSOs is growing. One of their goals is to cut out the middleman, i.e. the managed care organization, and negotiate directly with payers, whether corporations or the government, to provide care. Their logic is, "Why pay 20 percent to the HMO when we provide the care in any case and can do it directly?" Of course, managed care organizations point out that if PHOs are going to assume the role of insurance companies, they need to be regulated as insurance companies — including the need to have sufficient financial reserves. This may seem like a confusing business discussion, but it can have a very real effect on consumers. If, at some point in time, you have purchased health insurance through a PHO or PSO, you will need to make certain it is a financially sound organization. An insurance company without sufficient capital reserves to pay its bills is not good for consumers. This issue is still being discussed on federal and state levels and the legal structure needed to support the taking on of insurance risk by PHOs and PSOs has not yet been put in place, but it could happen in the near future.

Physician Practice Management (PPM) Companies

These companies, although relatively new on the health care scene, have grown in recent years primarily as a response to the new managed health care environment. With large networks of hospitals and managed care organizations being created through mergers, physicians have found they need to organize their own networks. They face the choice of being controlled by hospitals, being controlled by managed care, or controlling themselves. For many doctors, PPMs are the answer to this dilemma; some doctors are even turning to unions as a way of gaining negotiating strength.

PPMs operate in a number of ways: Some purchase physician practices, some help manage physician practices (including staff, billing, supplies etc.), and some only negotiate with managed care organizations on behalf of large numbers of physicians in loose networks. One of the primary goals of PPMs is to establish a large network of physicians to contract with managed care organizations. It makes a lot more sense for an

THE BLUE CROSS/BLUE SHIELD ASSOCIATION REPORTED THAT FOR THE FIRST TIME THE MAJORITY OF MEMBERS IN THE NATION'S 62 BLUE CROSS/BLUE SHIELD PLANS ARE NOW IN MANAGED CARE.

MCO to contract with a network of 500 physicians than it does to negotiate with 500 individual doctors. These networks may be comprised of doctors in a single specialty or different specialties (a multi-speciality group).

The above definitions may seem to be of little practical value at a time when your main concern is trying to determine who is going to provide your health care and how you will cope with a new system. These organizations, however, differ in ways which can impact your personal health care.

APPROXIMATELY

70 PERCENT OF

ALL HOSPITALS

HAVE MAN-

AGED CARE

CONTRACTS,

THE AMERICAN

HOSPITAL

ASSOCIATION

REPORTS.

•Issues and Controversy•

Mental Health

The provision of mental health services has lately become a major issue in managed care. It's not difficult to understand why.

If a person is physically ill or injured it's usually relatively easy, though not always, to identify the problem through examination and tests. When treatment is tendered, it's also fairly obvious when the person is better, although, clearly, full recovery may come in stages.

The problems of mental health are seldom so obvious, nor are the cures so well defined. Mental health is a spectrum, with variations from very sick to very healthy and everything in between. Most of us experience periods of extreme stress, depression, and other forms of behavior that, when they impair our ability to conduct our normal life activities effectively and with pleasure, could be defined as a mental health problem. With most physical disease or injury there is clearly a point when the patient is cured or at least managing the disease. That is not always true with emotional illness. The psychological counseling, psychotherapy, group therapies and other forms of treating mental health problems are time consuming, personnel intensive, expensive and accompanied by much debate about their effectiveness and outcomes.

In the days of indemnity insurance, patients could spend years in a therapeutic relationship, with their health insurance bearing all or most of the costs. That does not occur in managed care settings today.

HMOs, and sometimes state agencies, typically place restrictions on the number of visits to a mental health professional they will reimburse. They argue that if there is little or no evidence that someone who is treated on an inpatient basis for 60 days is "cured" any better than someone who is treated for only 30 days, it makes no sense to pay for an additional 30 days.

Of course, patients who have enjoyed a long-term relationship with a therapist, or those families who cannot cope with the behavior of one of their members and see hospitalization as either cure or respite, feel their needs are being ignored.

The political uproar has become so intense that the federal government passed a law requiring "full treatment" for mental health. Insurers and employers claim that such a requirement would vastly inflate health insurance costs and force cutbacks elsewhere. The impact of this regulation is not known because "full treatment" has yet to be clearly defined.

Most HMOs contract with a new kind of company that has emerged to serve the mental health needs of managed care members. Known as managed mental health or behavioral health companies, these firms contract with HMOs (usually on a capitated basis) to provide mental health services to their members. They focus on short-term inpatient and outpatient therapy. They avoid, if at all possible, the use of hospitals for inpatient therapy. Many HMOs have found that these companies do, in fact, control costs. Whether the outcomes of care are comparable is still an issue for debate.

Actually, many of these companies were formed before the rapid expansion of managed care because indemnity insurers were seeking ways to control the increasing costs of mental health care. Psychiatric hospitals have seen their occupancies plummet in recent years as the effect of these new systems took hold. While mental health professionals, and many of their patients, protest what they see as a lack of service (and employment), it is difficult to demonstrate a negative impact on the mental health of our nation or, specifically, on those enrolled in managed care.

Most managed care companies limit their coverages in this area, but some plans do have richer benefits than others. If this is an issue within a family, it is critical to scrutinize the benefit plan closely before selecting HMO coverage. Chapter 5 gives examples of the ranges of coverage and these examples can be used for comparison.

One thing MCOs try to strenuously avoid is over-hospitalization. That has occurred under indemnity plans. In fact, there are a number of significant lawsuits filed by patients against psychiatric hospitals where the patients and their families claim that the hospitals kept them hospitalized against their will in order to collect the insurance.

Highlights

Coverages, or benefits, offered by managed care plans differ greatly. It is important to assess coverages based on your personal or family health care needs. This chapter explains how to analyze coverages by using the simple chart we provide.

QUESTIONS ANSWERED IN THIS CHAPTER INCLUDE:

How do coverages in HMO plans compare?

What are some coverage issues to be sensitive to?

What is the range of HMO coverages?

Coverages

HOW TO GET WHAT YOU NEED

We all use health care differently. Some people may visit doctors frequently, others rarely. Some people are in and out of hospitals on a regular basis; some have never been hospitalized. Some people have chronic diseases that need to be followed and managed; some have no ongoing health problems. Some families are concerned about children and their needs, and others are concerned about the health issues associated with aging. In short, some health plans, because of their coverages (otherwise known as benefits), will better meet your needs than others. While cost, service, and quality will be important in this regard, it is really in the coverages offered that your individual needs are reflected.

Health plans vary widely in their coverages. Look at how you buy a car: If you have a large family, with passengers in the back seat all the time, then a four door vehicle is preferable. If you typically drive alone, then a two door car might suit your needs. You may opt for standard transmission or automatic drive. A powerful engine may be best for you, while someone else may desire economy.

Not only do most managed care organizations have a number of plans, but what an employer decides to purchase will influence the plans' design and coverages. A good example is dental or pharmacy benefits. Often employers may not include these coverages in their plans.

The best way to compare coverages is with a very systematic approach. To assist you in doing this we have created a structure for you. It will give you one method — and there are certainly others you can devise — to systematically compare health plans.

We reviewed over 50 different managed care plans and extracted examples of the coverages they offered. The following examples have been compiled to give you a sense of what constitutes minimal and substantial coverages. When comparing these "real life" examples with the coverages offered by a managed care organization you are considering, we suggest you rate each category on a scale of one to three. Since the needs of every individual and family differ, rate each coverage as it meets *your needs* and those of *your family*. Superior coverage that may not be important to you — for example, well-baby care for a single, non-parent — would not be rated highly.

We often assume that all managed care plans take care of every problem and to an unlimited extent. Not so! Be cautious — some treatments may not be covered by a managed care plan. These are known as exclusions and include such services as dental care, fertility treatment, elective surgery, experimental treatments and custodial care. Other benefits may be limited or "capped," such as a limit of 20 outpatient physical therapy visits or 20 visits to a psychiatrist or psychologist. Also, some plans may have a lifetime cap on the money spent for an individual's care — such as a million-dollar cap. Check on this, just as you would for an indemnity plan. A million dollars may sound like an astonishing sum, but it can be barely enough to cover extensive care for a serious problem.

The following pages describe a range of typical coverages offered by managed care plans. Each is accompanied by two examples. One example may be considered a "high-end" benefit and the other a "low-end" benefit. These examples can provide you with a point of reference to judge the quality of benefits offered by plans you are considering. However, remember that price is a consideration when comparing coverages, and usually the broader and more extensive the coverages, the greater the cost. Also, the HMOs you are considering may structure their coverages differently than these examples.

A SURVEY BY LANDMARK HEALTHCARE INC. SHOWED THAT OVER HALF THE MANAGED HEALTH PLANS SURVEYED COVERED SOME FORM OF ALTERNATIVE MEDICINE WITH ACUPUNCTURE (54 PERCENT), CHIROPRACTIC (45 PERCENT) AND MASSAGE THERAPY (25 PERCENT) BEING THE MOST FREQUENTLY COVERED.

Typical Coverages Offered By Managed Care Plans

Key: ▲ **High-End coverage**

▼ **Low-End coverage**

Allergy tests & treatments

▲ Routine coverage with copay

▼ $35 copay with testing

Alternative care (Acupuncture, Chiropractic care, Massage therapy, Naturopathy, Nutritionists & Dietitians, Yoga)

▲ Discounted rates through plan providers

▼ No coverage

Ambulance services

▲ 100% coverage

▼ 80% coverage out-of-network

Area of service

▲▼ Usually regional; some national or farther reaching networks offer care outside of area on a temporary or emergency basis

Consultations

▲▼ Usually covered as a regular office visit; copay often applies

Dental care

▲ Complete coverage for children under age 12

▼ No coverage available

Note: Those HMOs that do offer some form of dental coverage for adults do so through a rider provision.

Dependent definition

▲▼ Most often includes spouse up to age 65 and unmarried, dependent children up to age 19 if out of school or up to age 24 if full-time students

Diagnostic tests (CAT Scan, MRI, X-ray; Clinical laboratory)

▲   100% coverage when ordered by plan physician

▼   Copay for each test

Durable medical equipment

▲   100% coverage

▼   50% coverage

Ear & eye exams

▲   Routine coverage (as part of physical exam)

▼   Coverage only for those under age 18 or due to illness or injury

Note: Copay usually applies.

Emergency/urgent care

▲   100% coverage

▼   80% coverage

Note: Copay ranging from $35 to $100 can apply but is often waived if member is admitted to the hospital; an HMO may require prior notification before care is sought and care may have to be received at an affiliated facility.

Experimental treatment

▲ ▼   A very subjective area where HMOs are concerned. Most will not cover any treatment that has not been approved by the FDA

Extended care

▲   120 days per year

▼   25 days per year and/or $5,000 lifetime

Note: Most HMOs put a cap on the total amount spent annually or a life-time cap per member. Copays, ranging from $25 to $50 per day, often apply.

Family planning (Contraceptives, Elective abortion, Natural family planning, Tubal ligation, Vasectomy)

▲   100% coverage with copay

▼   Not covered

Note: Some HMOs require a deductible of up to $500 to be met before some of these services are covered.

Typical Coverages Offered By Managed Care Plans

Hearing aids

▲ ▼   Not covered

Home health care

▲   Up to 200 visits per year with copay

▼   Up to 20 visits per year

Note: HMOs often place a lifetime cap per member on this service ranging from $5,000 to $10,000.

Hospice care

▲   210 days per year with copay per visit

▼   125 days per year with copay per visit

Note: Some HMOs put a lifetime cap on the amount spent on hospice care per member, ranging from $5,000 to $10,000. Some require deductibles of up to $500 to be met before coverage commences.

Infertility

▲   Testing and prescriptions covered with copay

▼   Not covered

Note: While most HMOs will cover infertility treatments and some medications, they do not cover surgical procedures related to infertility.

Mammograms

▲   100% coverage

▼   Not covered

Maximum lifetime coverage

▲   Unlimited (except for those areas where specified otherwise, e.g., home health care, hospice care)

▼ $500,000 out-of-network coverage

Mental health - Inpatient

▲   Unlimited coverage in a hospital and 60 days annually in a psychiatric hospital

▼   30 days annually or 190 days lifetime

Mental health - Outpatient
▲   Unlimited coverage

▼   20 individual visits; 40 group visits per year

Note: Copay often applies.

Occupational therapy - Inpatient
▲   Unlimited

▼   60 days per year

Occupational therapy - Outpatient
▲   60 days per year

▼   20 days per year

Note: Copay often applies.

Organ transplants
▲ ▼   Usually includes corneal, bone marrow, kidney, and liver. In some cases, heart, lung, and pancreas are included.

Note: When covered, precertification is often necessary.

Out-of-network care
▲   80% coverage up to $500,000 lifetime cap

▼   Not covered

Note: When out-of-network care is permitted, HMOs often require a deductible of up to $1,000 to be met.

Outside second opinion
▲   80% coverage

▼   Not covered

Physical exams
▲   100% coverage for routine checkups

▼   Coverage only for exams due to illness or injury

Note: Some HMOs allow annual checkups for members through age 19 and over age 51 and include women's gynecological exams and Pap smears. These same HMOs often restrict exams to every five years for members 20-40 years old and every two years for those 41-50.

Typical Coverages Offered By Managed Care Plans

Physical therapy - Inpatient

▲ $500 per hospital stay

▼   30 days

Physical therapy - Outpatient

▲   90 visits per year

▼   20 visits per year

Note: Copay often applies.

Podiatry

▲   Complete coverage with copay

▼   Limited to surgical procedures

Pre-existing conditions

▲   Delay in coverage of 11 to 24 months after contract effective date

▼   Denial of coverage

Prenatal care (Including Amniocentesis, Chorionic Villi sampling, Ultrasound)

▲   100% coverage with copay per visit

▼   80% coverage after meeting $1,000 deductible for professional services; 80% coverage for hospital services

Prescription drugs

▲ $5 copay generic; $10 copay name brand

▼ $100 deductible for each family member; $300 family maximum

Prosthetics

▲   100% coverage

▼   50% coverage

Skilled nursing care

▲   365 days within 10 days of hospital discharge

▼   No coverage

Speech therapy - Inpatient

▲   Unlimited

▼   30 days coverage

Speech therapy - Outpatient

▲   90 visits per year

▼   20 visits per year

Note: Copay often applies.

Substance abuse - Inpatient

▲   Unlimited coverage

▼   30 days with 10% copay

Substance abuse - Outpatient

▲   Unlimited with copay

▼   30 visits annually after meeting $500 deductible

Surgery

▲   100% coverage

▼   80% coverage

Vision

▲▼   Usually covered as part of routine checkup or as related to illness but corrective eyeglasses or contact lenses are not covered

Well-baby care

▲▼   From birth to age two most HMOs provide 100% coverage for six visits annually (Some with copay); from ages two though 19, most cover annual visits.

Wellness programs

▲▼   Usually authorized and provided at no cost to members by the HMO. Can include a range of health education and health promotion services such as newsletters, resource guides, classes and courses. Some HMOs provide their members with discounted rates at health clubs and alternative care facilities.

In all managed care health plans, preventive care is supposed to be part of your coverages. When Paul Ellwood, MD, coined the term "health maintenance organization," the notion that costs could be controlled by reasonable preventive care was an integral element of the concept, as was eliminating wasteful and unnecessary care. But preventive care is not a benefit if you do not use it, and many HMOs have not done well in providing preventive care to their members. A good HMO should be aggressive in getting its members to utilize the preventive care offered. But if it fails in that responsibility, you should be assertive in utilizing it; you and your employer have paid for it! As a patient and a consumer, you need to be an active partner and assume responsibility for all aspects of your health care — prevention, cost, and quality.

OVER 90 PERCENT OF MANAGED CARE PLANS HAVE PHARMACY BENEFITS.

The purpose of this format is for you to rate the coverages offered by the health plan you are considering. This structure will assist you in making comparisons. The numerical totals should not be viewed as absolutes; rather they should serve as a guide for you in selecting a plan.

Rating - Rate each coverage: 3 = excellent, 2 = good, 1 = poor. Use the high end and low end examples, as well as coverages in other plans, as a guide to make these judgments.

Family Needs - Some coverages are more important to families than others. Rate the importance of this coverage to your family: 3 = very important, 2 = somewhat important, 1 = not important.

Multiply the rating by the family needs value to determine the total score for that coverage. Add up all the total scores to get the grand total for that HMO. **Example:**

Benefit	Rating of Coverage		Importance to Family		Total Score
PHYSICAL EXAMS	3	X	2	=	6

Plan Form

Plan Name_____

Benefit	Rating of Coverage		Importance to Family		Total Score
ALLERGY TESTS & TREATMENTS		X		=	
ALTERNATIVE CARE (ACUPUNCTURE CHIROPRACTIC CARE, MASSAGE THERAPY, NATUROPATHY, NUTRITIONISTS & DIETITIANS, YOGA)		X		=	
AMBULANCE SERVICES		X		=	
AREA OF SERVICE		X		=	
CONSULTATIONS		X		=	
DENTAL CARE		X		=	
DEPENDENT DEFINITION		X		=	
DIAGNOSTIC TESTS (CAT SCAN, MRI, X-RAY, CLINICAL LABORATORY)		X		=	
DURABLE MEDICAL EQUIPMENT		X		=	
EAR & EYE EXAMS		X		=	
EMERGENCY/URGENT CARE		X		=	
EXPERIMENTAL TREATMENT		X		=	
EXTENDED CARE		X		=	
FAMILY PLANNING (CONTRACEPTIVES, ELECTIVE ABORTION, NATURAL FAMILY PLANNING, TUBAL LIGATION, VASECTOMY)		X		=	

HEARING AIDS	X	=
HOME HEALTH CARE	X	=
HOSPICE CARE	X	=
INFERTILITY	X	=
MAMMOGRAMS	X	=
MAXIMUM LIFETIME COVERAGE	X	=
MENTAL HEALTH – INPATIENT	X	=
MENTAL HEALTH – OUTPATIENT	X	=
OCCUPATIONAL THERAPY – INPATIENT	X	=
OCCUPATIONAL THERAPY – OUTPATIENT	X	=
ORGAN TRANSPLANTS	X	=
OUT-OF-NETWORK CARE	X	=
OUTSIDE SECOND OPINION	X	=
PHYSICAL EXAMS	X	=
PHYSICAL THERAPY – INPATIENT	X	=
PHYSICAL THERAPY – OUTPATIENT	X	=
PODIATRY	X	=
PRE-EXISTING CONDITIONS	X	=
PRENATAL CARE (INCLUDING AMNIOCENTESIS, CHORIONIC VILLI SAMPLING, ULTRASOUND)	X	=
PRESCRIPTION DRUGS	X	=
PROSTHETICS	X	=
SKILLED NURSING CARE	X	=
SPEECH THERAPY – INPATIENT	X	=
SPEECH THERAPY – OUTPATIENT	X	=
SUBSTANCE ABUSE – INPATIENT	X	=
SUBSTANCE ABUSE – OUTPATIENT	X	=
SURGERY	X	=
VISION	X	=
WELL-BABY CARE	X	=
WELLNESS PROGRAMS	X	=

Grand Total _____

One very important issue when enrolling in any health plan, managed care or indemnity, is that of pre-existing conditions. It is critical to fully understand the health plan's policies on pre-existing conditions before you join. Many health insurance policies will not cover care for pre-existing conditions. A pre-existing condition is a health problem that you had *prior* to joining the plan. Examples of pre-existing conditions could include diabetes, asthma, or an injured back.

Some plans will exclude coverage completely and forever; others will cover them after a waiting period such as 60-120 days. It is important to be honest in answering questions about pre-existing conditions in health questionnaires. Hiding them could lead to loss of coverage when you need it most.

Federally qualified HMOs are not permitted to exclude care based on conditions or use waiting periods for employee groups larger than three. However, they may exclude care or use waiting periods in the case of smaller groups and individuals.

The time to understand what will be covered in your plan is *before* you enroll, not after you have enrolled, find you need care of a certain kind and then discover it is not covered.

Appendix A contains a copy of the chart that appeared on the previous pages. Permission is given to copy these pages; you may use them to rate each plan you are considering.

APPROXIMATELY 120 MILLION PEOPLE ARE COVERED BY MANAGED BEHAVIORAL HEALTH ORGANIZATIONS, ACCORDING TO THE NATIONAL COMMITTEE FOR QUALITY ASSURANCE.

•Issues and Controversy•

Poor Care

Some doctors, unfortunately, deliver poor care or make mistakes. This happens in managed care and it happens under indemnity insurance. When a doctor in an HMO makes a mistake, however, the whole organization gets blamed. This does not happen to indemnity insurers. They rarely get blamed for the mistakes the doctors make, primarily because they have had no role in selecting them or in influencing how they deliver care. The managed care organization does play that role, so it shares the blame.

Protect yourself by finding the best doctor you can and developing a long and trusting relationship. That is the best way to get good health care, whatever the system. If you do receive care that you believe is not up to standards you should use the grievance system of the health plan to address the issue. If the results of that process do not satisfy you, then go outside of the plan, to the local medical society, a consumer group, or the state agency that regulates HMOs (usually the insurance or health department). It is often helpful to have a second opinion in writing from a doctor not part of the plan to support your case. You will have to pay for it yourself, of course, but a doctor's judgment on a medical issue is worth far more than a layperson's.

Notes & Phone Numbers

_____

_____

_____

_____

_____

_____

_____

_____

_____

_____

_____

_____

_____

_____

_____

_____

_____

_____

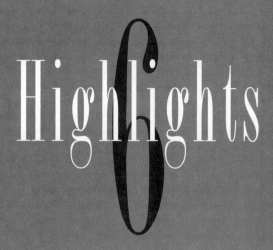

Highlights

Low costs and good coverages are the major reasons people join health plans. But while HMOs provide lower costs to members, there are still issues to watch out for, even in managed care.

QUESTIONS ANSWERED IN THIS CHAPTER INCLUDE:

Do HMO members pay anything at the doctor's office?

How do costs in HMOs differ from indemnity insurance?

What is a copay? a deductible?

How do I minimize my costs?

What do I pay if I go outside my plan?

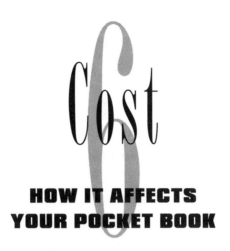

HOW IT AFFECTS
YOUR POCKET BOOK

This chapter is about the costs of managed care, to you and to your employer. If you are interested in how managed care controls costs, and how it has slowed the rapidly increasing costs of health care in our nation, be sure to read Chapter 8. Although some readers may not be interested in this "big picture" cost issue, it is important because the techniques used affect the way care is delivered and knowing these techniques will help you cope with the system and get the best care possible.

Initially, the concept of managed care was developed as a means of providing excellent quality of care at modest cost. The popularity of managed care and its tremendous growth, however, have had less to do with quality than with a focus on the cost of health care to employers and to our nation. But to most people, the cost of health care to the country is an irrelevant abstract. More relevant is the cost to an individual or a family. Of course, the cost to the country does influence and reflect personal cost because the expense of paying for the care of the nation's sick will be absorbed by every individual in higher premium prices, and/or taxes.

To an individual or family the two major aspects of the cost issue are: *(1) what the health plan costs an employer* and *(2) what it costs you.* If you are buying your own health insurance, these two aspects become a single concern.

A positive trend that has developed in many competitive health care markets is that individuals are now able to buy health insurance at rates that are not appreciably different than groups pay. This is a major change, brought about because of competition, and a real advantage for self-employed people and those employed by small firms. Of course, it is still easier and somewhat less expensive to be part of a large group, and that is why small businesses in many parts of the country are forming health insurance purchasing coalitions that bring together many small employers so they have the buying power of large groups. But people who are not healthy still have great difficulty buying health insurance if they are not part of a group plan.

There are two components that make up health insurance costs: (1) *basic premium costs* and (2) *deductibles and copayments*. When considering insurance, whether indemnity or managed care, you have to consider both.

The basic premium costs in HMOs vary depending on the plan and its benefits. A basic plan may cost from $150 to over $200 a month, per employee, depending on the coverages. Coverage for a family may range from $400 to over $600 per month. These amounts can vary by region of the country. Of course *your* costs will vary greatly depending on the portion your employer pays.

It is important to compare the deductibles, the copayments, and the premium costs with the coverages to determine value. A plan with extensive benefits (coverages) would be expected to cost more than a plan with lesser benefits.

Also, the monthly premium paid to an HMO could be higher than the premium charged by an indemnity insurer. To make a true cost comparison between the two you have to look at more than the premium.

A commercial health insurance plan, for instance, may include a $100 to $1,000 or higher annual deductible. Each year you must pay medical bills up to the level of the deductible before the insurance plan reimburses you for further medical expenses. HMOs rarely have deductibles. It is important to know this and to find out how much you must pay out-of-pocket before the plan starts paying.

In addition, most indemnity medical insurance covers 70 or 80 percent of eligible services; you pay the other 20 or 30 percent, generally up to a cap (a specified dollar limit). This is called co-insurance. Routine physical examinations, and often other preventive care including "well-baby care," are usually not covered by indemnity insurance. For hospitalization, HMOs generally cover all expenses, while many indemnity health insurance plans have ceilings on dollar payments and limits on the maximum number of days of hospitalization. Of course, HMOs are known for reducing hospital lengths of stay.

OVER HALF THE ANSWERERS POLLED BY LOUIS HARRIS AND ASSOCIATES WOULD LIKE TO SEE RATINGS ON HEALTH PLANS. FIFTY-EIGHT PERCENT WANTED CONSUMER RATINGS OF DOCTORS, AND 66 PERCENT WOULD LIKE TO SEE REPORT CARDS ON HOSPITALS.

CASE STUDY

Bill Raymond always had been active, running at least three or four times a week — until he tore the meniscus in his knee. Resigned to surgery, he arranged an appointment with an orthopedic surgeon known for his work in sports medicine. The doctor was not in Bill's HMO network, but Bill felt it would be worth the expense to have the surgery performed by someone he thought was the best. Since he was in a POS plan, Bill knew he had the option to go out of the network, though he would have to pay a larger share of the cost.

The surgery went well, but Bill was shocked to receive a bill amounting to thousands of dollars. Unfortunately, he had not received approval for the surgery from his health plan. Because the surgeon was not in the plan, the hospital and the anesthesiologist, who were both in the plan, were treated as out-of-plan providers and Bill had to bear a substantial portion of their fees. ∎

Deductibles and copayments also are very important to consider. A deductible is the amount you must pay first, before your insurance starts paying. How high is it — $200, $500, $2,500? Whatever it is, it will come out of your pocket, so allow for it when deciding what to pay for your plan. Also, you need to keep track of it so when you reach your individual or family deductible you don't make the mistake of paying more. A typical deductible might be $250 per individual or $500 for a family. When an individual has spent $250 or a family $500 in combined expenses the limit would be reached and they would not have to pay any more.

A copay is the dollar amount you pay each time you use a service that qualifies for coverage. If you are going to use a particular service regularly — say, physical therapy — you will want to consider how much your copayments will amount to. Many plans carry a $15 to $25 copayment for some services each time they are used. They may also "cap" or limit the number of visits each year. How will that affect you? Also, copayments do not count towards deductible limits.

Examine the premium. Examine the deductibles and copayments. Calculate how much it is likely to cost you based on the way you and your family use health care.

One of the most important factors in keeping your costs low is following the rules of the HMO. Do not seek services without authorization. Use in-network providers whenever possible. Complete all paperwork when required. Be certain to get approvals when necessary.

All of these techniques can help you control costs and avoid hassles!

Most important, do not assume that all HMOs take care of every medical problem to an unlimited extent. Some treatments may *not* be covered by an HMO. Be alert as you consider your choices in any type of managed care plan. Check on the extent of your coverages, just as you would for an indemnity plan.

If you are in a Point of Service plan (POS) do not assume you can simply go outside the plan's network of providers whenever you want and submit a bill and have 70 or 80 percent of it reimbursed. POS plans, sometimes labeled "freedom plans" or "HMOs without walls," may have complex rules to follow. You may still need prior approval for certain procedures, such as surgery, or for tests. If you choose a non-participating provider (a doctor not in the plan) you may find your-self paying the hospital bill even if the hospital is part of the HMO network. Or you may find the plan treats the anesthesiologist as being outside the plan, even if he is in it, if the surgeon is not part of the plan network. Be certain to notify the plan, or seek approval, as required by the plan's policies. POS plans shift a great deal of responsibility to the individual. Make certain you understand the HMO's policies and talk to the member services staff at the plan to maximize your coverages and choices while you minimize your costs.

Also, finding out how much it will cost you to go out-side the plan, if you choose, can be difficult and time

THIRTY-NINE PERCENT OF THOSE SURVEYED BY THE EMPLOYEE BENEFIT RESEARCH INSTITUTE AND THE GALLUP ORGANIZATION INC. SAID THEY WOULD PAY FOR A MEDICAL TEST THEMSELVES, IF THEIR DOCTOR RECOMMENDED IT, EVEN IF THEIR HEALTH INSUR-ANCE WOULD NOT PAY FOR IT.

consuming, so make sure you plan ahead. In fact, planning ahead is often essential because many POS plans require 10-14 days (or even longer) prior notification for approval to use out-of-network providers — or they will not pay any part of the bill.

POS PLAN EXAMPLE

DOCTOR'S FEE: $1000

POS PAYMENT
USUAL &
CUSTOMARY: $750

80% OF USUAL
& CUSTOMARY: $600

PLAN PAYS: $600
PATIENT PAYS: $400

Determining how much you will pay to go outside of the plan requires direct conversation with the managers of your health plan. You need to understand the percentage you will pay — 80 percent, for example. But 80 percent of what? It is unlikely to be 80 percent of the doctor's bill. Rarely do insurance companies pay that rate. More typically they will pay a percentage of the plan's fee, or a percentage of "usual, customary and reasonable," a common term in indemnity plans. Try to find out what the plan's fee is or what is usual, customary and reasonable in your area *before* you go out of the network.

Whether an HMO costs you and your family less than a traditional insurance plan may depend on how much you use medical services. In most cases, however, you should save money since there are so few out-of-pocket expenses. The premium — often paid totally or partially by your employer — should cover most of your treatment.

If you belong to a federally qualified plan and your employer pays all or a part of the premium, the employer contribution must be at least equal to the amount contributed to the principal health insurance plan offered by the company. Also, if you pay a share of the cost, your employer must give you the opportunity to have your share deducted from your paycheck. One thing is certain: Managed care should lower your out-of-pocket costs and simplify your method of payment.

When Your Health Plan Refuses To Pay

As has been pointed out, not all health plans cover every kind of care, and they will not pay for services they don't cover. They also may not pay if the care is provided in violation of their policies; for example, if you go to a specialist without prior authorization. Other common areas of dispute are emergency care, nursing home care, ambulance service, and hospital bills.

Sometimes there is disagreement between members and health plans over payment. This could be caused by an administrative error on the health plan's part, or it could be caused by a lack of understanding on the part of the member — or even the doctor — of the HMO's policies. It could be a difference of opinion between a doctor and the HMO about what care was appropriate. A good example is the issue of "off-label" drug uses. Many doctors use certain drugs for a purpose different than that for which they were initially approved. This is common and it is not illegal or inappropriate. However, many plans will not reimburse for such "off-label" uses. A Gallup poll of oncologists stated that one of every eight patients cared for by these specialists belonged to a plan that would not cover "off-

EMPLOYERS PAY ABOUT THREE-QUARTERS OF HEALTH CARE COSTS FOR EMPLOYEES, ACCORDING TO A STUDY BY *BUSINESS AND HEALTH* MAGAZINE.

label" uses. If your plan does not, it could mean you would end up paying for a drug, even though you and your doctor thought it would be, or should be, covered.

Payment: Important Points to Consider

How much is deducted from your paycheck each month for health insurance?

How much do you pay for an office visit to the doctor?

If you are treated by a doctor not participating in the plan, how much do you pay?

What do you pay for drugs and medications?

What are the procedures and time frame for reimbursement of any out-of-pocket expenses?

If non-network doctors bill for service, do they bill you directly or do they bill the plan?

What is the total amount you must pay before you reach your deductible limit?

Is there a dollar limit on any benefits, such as a maximum of $6,000 a year with $30,000 lifetime maximum for mental health benefits?

What does the plan cost each month for individuals? for families?

When was the last premium increase?

How do recent increases compare with other managed care plans and other insurance plans offered by your employer?

What will your employer's contribution be and is that contribution the same for all health plans offered?

If you must use a non-plan hospital in an emergency, how quickly must you file a claim and how long on average will you have to wait for reimbursement?

What are the penalties for not reporting emergency admissions according to plan guidelines?

If you disagree with a bill from your health plan, you should follow these following steps to resolve it.

1. *Call the plan and discuss the issue with a service representative. Be certain to keep a written record of the date and time of the call, the name of the representative, and his or her response.*

2. *If the issue is not resolved, get the name of the person to whom you should write and send him or her a letter fully explaining the issue, accompanied by copies of any documentation you have.*

3. *If your claim is still denied, follow the plan's grievance process (see p. 105).*

4. *If you cannot get satisfaction from the plan, write the state insurance department, again explaining fully and including copies of any documentation you have, and a complete description of the plan's response.*

•Issues and Controversy•

"Drive-through Births"

This issue, as well as some others, derive from two shared characteristics of managed care: First, managed care attempts to reduce unnecessary costs and especially the use of hospitals; second, managed care is not always sensitive to how cost-reduction efforts, however well-intended, will be perceived by the public.

"Drive-through Births" is a term some of the media used to describe a policy some HMOs adopted that limited a woman's stay in the hospital after giving birth to a single day. While it is true that for many women and their newborns a single postpartum day may be adequate, or even "best" because hospitals carry their own risks, for some mothers one day is not enough. The perception that HMOs were pushing mothers and babies out of the hospital before they were ready was a public relations disaster, literally against "God, motherhood and apple pie"! State and federal legislatures rushed to defend motherhood (What more noble cause?) and bills were submitted to state legislatures across the country to ban such policies. Most required 48 hours hospital stay for vaginal deliveries and 96 hours for Caesarean sections.

Congress then jumped into the act with a bill called the "Newborns and Mothers Health Protection Act of 1995."

What sympathizers of all these bills failed to recognize is that some mothers may want to leave the hospital as soon as possible, perhaps in less than a day, and that many mothers do not even want to go to a hospital to give birth but prefer birthing centers. These bills and requirements would also cost consumers and businesses additional millions in health care costs, many of them unnecessary. Managed care organizations, of course, quickly backed off the policies limiting births to one hospital day and adopted the more reasonable posture that decisions on discharge were better left to doctors and patients, which is how it should be.

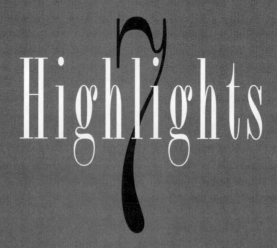

Highlights

Quality is a major concern of consumers. No one wants second rate health care. This chapter will help you judge quality in an HMO.

QUESTIONS ANSWERED IN THIS CHAPTER INCLUDE:

What are the pro and con views on quality in managed care?

What is accreditation? How important is it?

How do I find out if my health plan is accredited?

What does it mean if a health plan is federally qualified?

What should I look for in doctors and hospitals from a health plan?

What are outcomes? How important are they?

How can I check on the quality of an HMO?

How can I use "report cards" on HMOs to make better choices?

What do I look for to judge the quality of service in an HMO?

How do I deal with complaints I have about service or quality?

Can I sue an HMO?

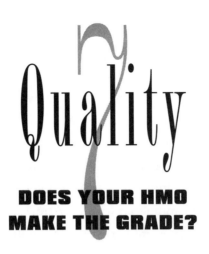

Quality

DOES YOUR HMO MAKE THE GRADE?

Quality is especially important in managed care because the plan doesn't just pay for your medical care; it is actually *providing* your health care. While the goal of this chapter is to provide you with an outline for comparing one HMO with another, the question of quality is also raised when people discuss HMOs as compared with traditional indemnity insurance.

Despite the concerns voiced by some critics, and the horror story headlines you may occasionally read, the predominance of evidence to date suggests that enrollees in HMOs, or other kinds of managed care plans, receive the same quality of health care as people covered by traditional indemnity insurance. There is some debate on the impact of managed care on people with chronic illnesses, but many managed care plans are addressing those needs with special programs. For example, Oxford Health Care, a leading East Coast HMO, has developed specialty care teams to deal with chronic illnesses such as diabetes, asthma and heart disease.

The supporters of HMOs believe that managed care can improve quality through its emphasis on prevention and coordination of care. There is evidence to support this. A KPMG Peat Marwick study demonstrated that in areas where there is a high level of managed care, mortality rates were eight percent less than predicted, while in areas with a low level of managed care they were two percent lower than predicted. *U.S. News and World Report* cited examples of managed care systems that demonstrated care and prevention results exceeding national averages. For example, in the three HMOs they used as comparisons, the mammography rates were 71 percent, 84 percent and 55 percent compared to a national average of 33 percent. The pediatric immunization rates were 92 percent, 95 percent and 87 percent as compared to a national average of 56 percent. A study in the *Journal of the American Medical Association (JAMA)* showed that mortality rates for people with hypertension were lower in HMOs than in fee-for-service plans. The same study showed equivalent positive results for diabetic patients.

In an October 1996 *JAMA* editorial on managed care, George D. Lundberg, M.D., the editor of *JAMA*, and Paul Ellwood, M.D., often referred to as the "father" of the HMO, concluded, "Despite anecdotes, some lurid, we have no objective evidence of any overall decline in the system. It has contained costs, it provides easily accessible comprehensive care to its insured and, on the whole, it has not yet jeopardized quality."

This statement does not deny the existence of problems and incidents of harm to patients by poor decisions and/or policies, but, on the whole, managed care competes well on the quality front.

Clearly, final results are not in and the measuring of

outcomes (the results of care and treatment) will continue. Despite the individual complaints (many of them justified) about long waits to get appointments, the difficulty of getting referrals to specialists, and the occasionally dramatic stories of denial of treatment, most studies of large populations conclude "no difference" or "positive results in favor of managed care" when it comes to measuring the quality of care delivered by managed health plans.

Yet, there are still many people who believe managed care is bad and that any effort to control immediate and unrestricted access to care is a terrible thing. The horror stories we hear and read are not untrue. They may be isolated incidents, or they may be acute warning signs of problems within the system. As such, they should be used to prompt examination and review, so that system faults can be corrected. These days the efforts of many large employers and government, both of whom have embraced managed care, are focused on working with their managed care providers to measure and improve care rather than turning to other options. For most of us, this means dealing with the system we have and working to improve it.

There are four dimensions of quality to be considered in the process of selecting the best managed care program for you and your family: (1) *accreditation*, (2) *provider network*, (3) *service*, and (4) *outcomes*, including consumer satisfaction.

A HARVARD SCHOOL OF PUBLIC HEALTH/HARRIS POLL REPORTED THAT MORE MEMBERS OF MANAGED CARE PLANS (22 PERCENT) FELT THEY HAD PROBLEMS GETTING NEEDED TREATMENT THAN DID PATIENTS COVERED BY FEE-FOR- SERVICE INSURANCE (15 PERCENT).

Accreditation

Like hospitals, HMOs and other managed care organizations may be accredited.

The importance of accreditation is that you know an objective third party has assessed the organization by a set of pre-determined standards. Accreditation tends to focus on process, rather than outcomes. However, the press for outcomes measurement undoubtedly will be a future emphasis of accreditation. (The issue of outcomes is examined in greater detail later in this chapter.)

Given a choice between an accredited and unaccredited HMO, you know the accredited HMO has met specific standards. Large employers have recognized the value of accreditation and some will consider only accredited HMOs as part of their health plan.

There are several organizations that offer accreditation to managed care organizations: The National Committee for Quality Assurance (NCQA), the Joint Commission on the Accreditation of Healthcare Organizations (JCAHO), the Accreditation Association for Ambulatory Health Care (AAAHC), and the American Accreditation and Healthcare Commission (AAHCC), formerly known as the Utilization Review Accreditation Commission (URAC). The AAAHC was spun off of the JCAHO in 1979. The AAHCC, while focusing primarily on HMOs, now accredits PPOs as well, having acquired the American Accreditation

Program, Inc. which was the only organization to accredit PPOs.

However, of the four accrediting bodies, the NCQA and the JCAHO dominate the field.

The NCQA

The NCQA has developed 50 standards for accrediting managed care organizations which fall into six categories: quality management and improvement, physician credentialing, members' rights and responsibilities, preventive health services, medical records and utilization management.

Managed care organizations may apply for accreditation by asking for a survey based on the criteria outlined in the Standards of Accreditations. Experienced managed care professionals, including doctors, make up the survey team. Under the NCQA standards, four levels of accreditation can be achieved:

1. *Full accreditation for three years*

2 *1-year accreditation*

3. *Provisional accreditation*

4. *Denial*

EIGHTY-TWO PERCENT OF MANAGERS SURVEYED BY THE INTERNATIONAL FOUNDATION OF EMPLOYEE BENEFIT PLANS DESCRIBED THE TOPIC OF HEALTH PLAN QUALITY AS VERY IMPORTANT AMONG HEALTH BENEFIT ISSUES. ONE QUARTER THOUGHT QUALITY WAS MORE IMPORTANT THAN COST.

Of the approximately 660 HMOs in the country, about 330, or 50 percent, have sought NCQA accreditation. Of these, 118 have received full NCQA accreditation, 85 have received one-year accreditation, 24 have received provisional accreditation, 25 have been denied accreditation, 18 reviews are pending, and 59 reviews are scheduled. Of the approximately 60 to 65 million Americans enrolled in managed care plans, 28 million are in HMOs that have sought NCQA accreditation. With the urging of the Robert Wood Johnson Foundation, which funded much of the early work in this area, HMO accreditation is on its way to achieving the same high standards as those used for hospitals. In fact, some employers now require that a plan have NCQA accreditation before offering it to their employees. The NCQA also accredits other forms of managed care including POS plans, group HMOs, staff HMOs, IPAs and mixed models.

Summary reports of those plans that have been accredited by the NCQA, and an accreditation status list that catalogs all plans that have sought NCQA accreditation are updated monthly and are available to the public. They can be obtained by contacting the NCQA at its customer service number, (800) 839-6487, or by writing to the NCQA at P.O. Box 533, Annapolis Junction, MD 20701-0533. Full reports are $3.00 apiece and must be prepaid. Summaries of an HMO's accreditation status also can be obtained by visiting the NCQA website at http://NCQA.org.

The JCAHO

The Joint Commission on Accreditation of Healthcare Organizations, the organization best know for accrediting hospitals, began accrediting "networks" in 1994. Network accreditation focuses on the following key performance areas:

1. *Preventive care.*

2. *The continuum of care.*

3. *The credentialing and performance of doctors, nurses and other staff*

4. *The rights of patients*

5. *The procedures in place for measuring and improving the quality of patient care*

6. *Education and communication*

7. *Network leadership*

8. *Management of information*

The Joint Commission examines services provided by networks through ambulatory settings, home care, hospitals, laboratories, long-term care, and mental health.

The Commission follows the same model for accreditation decisions that it uses in hospitals: accreditation with commendation; accreditation with recommendations for improvement; conditional accreditation; pre-

A STUDY BY NATIONAL RESEARCH CORPORATION SHOWED THAT 22.9 PERCENT OF HMO ENROLLEES WERE NOT ABLE TO GET REFERRALS TO SPECIALISTS AS COMPARED TO 6.1 PERCENT IN FEE-FOR-SERVICE PLANS.

liminary non-accreditation; denied accreditation. Since 1994, when the JCAHO first began accrediting managed care organizations, it has granted accreditation to 16, and is currently reviewing 20 more applications.

Consumers who wish to know if a plan is accredited by the JCAHO and the status of that accreditation can call the JCAHO's customer service number (630) 792-5000. Performance reports for all of the health care organizations accredited by the Joint Commission which include hospitals, psychiatric and long-term care facilities, substance abuse programs, community mental health programs, and home care as well as managed care networks can be obtained at no cost by calling that number. The JCAHO has these reports available at its website (http://www.jcaho.org).

Since relatively few managed care organizations are currently accredited (approximately half of the 660 plus plans) it is clear that accreditation is still a new and not widely accepted concept. Nonetheless, 19 million people, or 42 percent of the population enrolled in managed care are members of the over 300 managed care plans that have been reviewed. Of course, there is no accreditation for indemnity health plans because they do not deliver health care, they only pay for it.

Federal Government Qualification

A similar process to accreditation is federal qualification. HMOs that are federally qualified have been judged by the Office of Managed Care of the Health Care Financing Administration (HCFA) to meet certain basic standards of operation. An HMO must apply for qualification from the HCFA, which then visits the facility and considers such factors as health services delivery, availability, accessibility, quality assurance, financial stability, and marketing procedures before granting qualification. Qualification, which may take several months, is a one-time process, unless an HMO is not initially approved and wishes to apply for approval at a later date. HMOs that are qualified are not subject to requalification. Hence, it is a good idea to find out how long an HMO has been federally qualified. The more recent the qualification, the better the chances the HMO is still up to par. With the relaxation of federal qualification standards in 1982, HMOs today are less likely to pursue federal qualification. As a result it has become a less significant standard in recent years.

Provider Network

Although managed care organizations use other kinds of providers such as dentists, podiatrists, nurses, chiropractors, physical therapists and pharmacies, it is primarily the quality of doctors and hospitals that are of concern to most people. The following list of questions will assist you in assessing these providers. You should seek well-trained, board certified physicians and fully

DATA COMPILED AND REPORTED BY *U.S. NEWS AND WORLD REPORT* SHOWED THAT GOOD MANAGED CARE SYSTEMS REDUCED CAESAREAN SECTIONS AND LOW BIRTH WEIGHT IN PREMATURE NEWBORNS AND INCREASED MAMMOGRAPHY RATES AND PEDIATRIC IMMUNIZATION RATES AS COMPARED TO NATIONAL AVERAGES.

accredited hospitals of good reputation. These should be the most important factors, in addition to coverages, in your selection. Typically HMOs are quite careful in their selection of physicians. Frequently, they will mandate board certification. They should also review hospital appointments, malpractice history, office hours, coverage arrangements when the doctor is not available, and do site visits to check out the doctors' office facilities and even their record keeping. These are all things a good HMO will do.

The following are some questions you should ask about the provider network:

Doctors

Is there a sufficient number of primary care doctors
from which to choose and are they accessible to you?

On what hospital staff is the doctor you are selecting?
If you're hospitalized, it will probably be there.

What are the qualifications of the plan's doctors? What percentage are
board certified? (Seek a minimum of 80 percent.)

Can you choose your primary care doctor or are you assigned one?
Can each family member have a different primary care physician?

Can you change primary care doctors once you have chosen one?
How difficult is it? How often can you change?

Are you given or can you request a list of the plan's doctors with
information on their education and training?
Are the doctors in whom you are interested still accepting patients?

Are they pleased with the HMO and planning to continue the relationship?

Do others beside your primary physician, such as nurse practitioners
or physician's assistants, handle routine visits and examinations?

Must you use only those specialists affiliated with the plan?
Must you get a second opinion within the plan or can you
go outside the plan for a second opinion? What is the cost of this?

Must your primary care doctor refer you to a specialist? What is the process?
How long is the typical waiting period for an appointment?

If you have a chronic disease, can a specialist in that disease
serve as your primary care physician?

Doctors

Is there an adequate number of specialists and subspecialists in the network?

If you are referred to a specialist does one referral last for an extended period (6-12 months) or do you need a new referral for each visit?

Is your primary physician involved in your care if you are hospitalized?

If it is an IPA model, are the doctors you would select relatively close by?

What provisions, if any, are made for evening, weekend, and emergency care?

What provisions, if any, are made for care when you are away from home?

An HMO's network of hospitals is obviously a very critical aspect of its provider strength. Despite this, many people, perhaps in the belief they will never be hospitalized, ignore looking thoroughly into the hospital network.

Reviewing the list of hospitals in the HMO provider directory is not enough. Although a large number of hospitals may be listed you may not have access to all of them. Typically, the hospital that will be your primary admitting hospital for most problems that require hospitalization will be dependent on (1) *where you live* or (2) *where your primary care doctor has a medical staff appointment*. Call the HMO and ask what determines where you will be hospitalized if it is necessary and if you have any choices. One other issue that comes into play in determining where you may be hospitalized is the type of contract the HMO has with the hospital. It may be based only on a specific number of patient days, or a set number of patients or, more critically, on one or two particular services.

For example, a hospital may have a contract only for obstetrics and pediatrics. Another hospital may be under contract just for cardiology and open heart surgery. If you believe you may need to be hospitalized for a critical problem, find out in advance where you would be hospitalized, and be certain it is a hospital with a good reputation.

When you join an HMO ask if all the hospitals are available to you and/or under what conditions. Some HMO members have found themselves traveling 30-40 miles to a hospital because their HMO did not have a contract with one closer or because closer hospitals were contracted only for selected services. Of course, if you live in a rural area, or if the hospital you have to drive to is a truly excellent one, that may not be an issue.

Many HMOs advertise their "centers of excellence" programs. Usually this means the HMO has contracted with one hospital for a particular tertiary care service, such as transplants or cardiothoracic (open-heart) surgery. Hospitals make these agreements and give the HMOs substantial price discounts in exchange for the volume the HMO generates. However, it's useful to try

> PATIENTS WITH LOWER BACK PAIN IN HMOS HAVE EQUAL OUTCOMES WITH LOWER UTILIZATION ACCORDING TO A STUDY PUBLISHED IN THE *NEW ENGLAND JOURNAL OF MEDICINE.*

to determine if the "center of" excellence was selected for its excellence or for its prices! Is the hospital really noted for its excellence in that procedure or for that care, or are there "more excellent" programs around? If you can, talk to health professionals you know and ask about the hospital's reputation for that service, or ask the HMO or the hospital if they have comparative data. You should find out if the program is accredited by, or has been recognized by, a specialty accrediting group. For example, the American College of Radiology will tell you if a hospital has an accredited mammography program.

Few of us plan to have transplants or open-heart surgery, and when we do need that kind of care it is often under such great time and emotional pressure we can't deal with the issue in such a rational manner. However, if you believe you or a member of your family may need some kind of special care because of a chronic condition, it is wise to check the resources available in the HMO before you join, rather than at the critical moment you need them.

One of the best sources for information on hospitals is the Joint Commission on Accreditation of Healthcare Organizations, the major accrediting body for hospitals.

The Joint Commission examines such things as: patient care function; service providers and staff; physical environment and safety; and organizational leadership and management.

Only about one percent of the hospitals are denied accreditation, with the result that the Joint Commission has often been accused of being too lenient. On the other hand, denying a hospital accreditation is tantamount to closing it and is not a decision to be taken lightly. Despite these criticisms, the JCAHO remains the "gold standard" of hospital accreditation.

If a hospital is not accredited by the JCAHO you should make certain it is accredited by the appropriate state agency. You can contact your state department of health to obtain a copy of the accreditation report. Some hospitals, especially smaller ones, may avoid the expense of JCAHO accreditation if the state they are located in has a comprehensive accreditation process.

Typically, a hospital will publish its accreditation status. You can ask the hospital or call the Joint Commission. The Joint Commission's accreditation reviews are available in writing by contacting the Joint Commission at (630) 792-5000 or on the internet at http://www.jcaho.org.

A CARE DATA SURVEY OF MANAGED PLAN MEMBERS SHOWED THAT 70 PERCENT OF THOSE POLLED WERE SATISFIED WITH THE QUALITY OF HOSPITALS WHILE 52 PERCENT WERE SATISFIED BY THE CONCERN SHOWN FOR THEIR WELL-BEING.

Following are some questions you should ask about the hospitals in any health plan you are considering:

Hospitals

Does the managed care plan utilize more than one hospital?

Are the hospitals relatively close by and readily accessible?
Are they accredited by the JCAHO?

What is the reputation of the hospital in the community?
Does it have excellent medical and nursing staffs?

If you have a chronic disease are there hospitals in the plan with special expertise in that area? Can you select a PCP or a specialist on that medical staff as your primary care physician?

What is the quality and scope of services offered?
Do they have tertiary services such as burn care, or open-heart surgery?

Of course, providers other than doctors and hospitals are important to your health care. When considering a health plan be sure to have answers to the following questions, especially for those services that are important to you:

Other Providers

Does the HMO have a pharmacy benefit?
If so, is it mail order or at local stores?
If it is at local pharmacies, is there at least one close to your home?

Is long-term care part of the plan?
If so, what long-term facilities are part of the network?

Are dental, chiropractic, podiatry and physical therapy covered?
If so, is there a reasonable number of practitioners in your area?
Are they ones you know or can
you assure yourself they are of good reputation?

Quality of Care – Outcomes

Ideally, the way we should judge the quality of any health care provider — doctor, hospital or HMO — is on the results of their care. Does the care have the intended or best possible result? The results of care are called "outcomes" and studies to track and measure the results are called outcomes studies.

"Outcomes" is one of the buzz words in health care

these days. Major employers and the government are demanding outcomes studies so they can judge the cost effectiveness of the care they are paying for and patients are receiving. Professional groups like the American Medical Association (AMA) and medical specialty groups are encouraging outcomes studies to develop what are known as clinical practice guidelines, sometimes called "best practices," so physicians and hospitals can deliver the best, most effective care. HMOs are also important leaders in outcomes studies because they have hundreds of doctors treating thousands of patients and good information systems to keep track of the care and its results. HMOs have the potential to make major contributions in this important field. Some do, but many do not, primarily because of the lack of good clinical information systems.

With outcomes data, consumers, as well as employers and the government, could make choices of providers based on results. While that is an admirable goal, and for the government and large employers it is becoming a reality, it will be many years before such information is widely available to consumers in a way it can be used.

One serious effort to measure quality in health plans is the National Committee on Quality Assurance (NCQA) *Quality Compass*. The *Quality Compass* includes detailed data on quality measures drawn from the NCQA Health Employer Data and Information Set (HEDIS), a set of measures that the NCQA has available on 226 health plans nationwide.

HEDIS is comprised of data reflecting clinical performance in such measures as childhood immunizations, cholesterol screening, the weight of newborns (an indication of good prenatal care), mammography screenings and management of chronic diseases such as asthma and diabetes.

Available on a CD-ROM or in print, regional reports cost $500 (print), or the entire database can be purchased for $3,200.

The report enables purchasers of health care to compare the quality of one plan to another using these measures. Unfortunately, it is expensive, and will likely be used primarily by large employers. Also, many of the nation's largest health plans declined to share their data with the NCQA. Ultimately, however, the NCQA very probably will require participation in HEDIS as a part of accreditation.

Some true outcomes data are available to consumers. New York State, for example, has tracked the results of hospitals and individual doctors in terms of the survival rates of their patients after cardiac bypass surgery. Any potential patient can now check the results of a surgeon and hospital before making a choice.

HMOs often publish "report cards" on their care, but the results published tend to be more measures of the process of care, or satisfaction ratings by members,

OF EMPLOYERS WITH 10,000 OR MORE EMPLOYEES, 59 PERCENT USE HEDIS TO MEASURE QUALITY IN HEALTH PLANS. IN CONTRAST, 25 PERCENT OF THOSE WITH 1,000 TO 9,999 EMPLOYEES AND ONLY SIX PERCENT WITH FEWER THAN 1,000 USE HEDIS, ACCORDING TO A WATSON WYATT WORLDWIDE STUDY.

rather than medical outcomes. Information on the percentage of children receiving appropriate and timely vaccinations, or the percentage of women having annual pap smears, or the percentage of diabetics receiving foot care, is very important and affects the quality of care, but is not a true outcomes study.

Where an HMO has, and will make available, outcomes studies, consumers should request and review these to see how the HMO compares to its competition on the care measured by the study. If outcomes studies are not available, review whatever report cards are available. Those that measure satisfaction are also important because they will give you a sense of how the HMO's members feel about the quality of care and service. In fact, some HMOs — Aetna/U.S. Healthcare, for example — publish member ratings of individual doctors that are available for review.

HMO Quality Checks

When you want to check on the quality of your health plan, managed care or indemnity, call your state health or insurance department (listed in Appendix B) and ask if they have reports on:

Complaints – Many states maintain records of complaints made against insurers. Try to find out the number of complaints per one thousand members, or the number of complaints unresolved, or the number of complaints resolved against the HMO. The ratio per thousand members is important because a large HMO is likely to receive more complaints than a small one. The reports of some states will have all of this calculated for you.

Disenrollment Figures – The percentage of members each year who decide to change plans may be indicative of service or other problems in an HMO. Nationally the average is about 20 percent per year for voluntary changes (an involuntary change could entail an employer changing plans). Inquire to see if your state maintains these figures for any plan you are considering. It is useful to compare the percentage of plan turnover with other plans in the community. If the turnover or disenrollment rate of a plan is much higher than others, it would be worthwhile to find out why.

Medical Loss Ratios – As an indicator of quality, medical loss ratios are less valid than plan turnover or complaint ratios. The medical loss ratio is the amount of money, expressed as a percentage of total revenue, that a plan spends on medical care. The remaining percentage is spent on overhead and, in the case of for-profit organizations, profit.

Many for-profit HMOs have medical loss ratios in the high seventies and low eighties. Some not-for-profit HMOs have medical loss ratios in the low to mid-nineties. Unfortunately, spending more money on care does not always indicate good quality. An HMO may have a medical loss ratio in the seventies because it is well run and efficient while an HMO of poorer quality may have a medical loss ratio in the nineties because it

A SURVEY BY THE COMMON-WEALTH FUND FOUND THAT WOMEN IN HMOS WERE MORE LIKELY TO RECEIVE PREVENTIVE SERVICES THAN WOMEN IN NON-HMO INSURANCE PLANS.

is badly run. However, the medical loss ratio, if vastly different — either higher or lower — than other plans, may be a signal to investigate further.

Financial Stability – Knowing that your health plan is on sound financial footing is important. You don't want to be in a plan that can't pay its bills to doctors and hospitals. Some HMOs are known for paying providers slowly. That could be the result of the challenges of rapid growth, or it could be that they want to hold on to premium payments as long as possible to earn the interest — or it could be a sign of financial difficulty.

If an HMO is large, well established, and its plans are used by prominent employers in your area, you can be pretty sure it is financially stable. For a more specific assessment, call the state insurance department and ask if they have fiscal soundness ratings available.

Doctor Turnover – This relates to doctors who are leaving the plan. Although it is hard to obtain statistics on this, you can do a little research on your own. Ask the HMO what their turnover rate is. Ten percent annually is reasonable. If they don't have or won't supply you with that information, call a number of doctors listed and ask the office staff if they still participate in the plan. If they respond no, ask why. You may get some interesting insights into the plan's relationship with its doctors and you also can gain a sense of how accurate the plan's roster of providers is. Some plans continue to list doctors who have left because it enhances the appearance of their network. This can be especially important if you are choosing a plan because a particular doctor is in it. Call the doctor's office first, before you make a commitment!

Service

The term service broadly encompasses all aspects of the HMO as it delivers care to its members.

Service is more important than ever to consumers. In many metropolitan areas, as managed care grows and enrolls more members, health plans sign on more doctors and hospitals. As a result, the physician and hospital networks of plans become more similar and quality less distinguishable: One provider's network can look pretty much the same as any other competitor's network. This leaves quality in service as an important way to choose among managed care plans. Health care plans realize this, and that is why the new emphasis is on quality; many consumers perceive service as being strongly related to quality.

And service quality is strongly related to medical quality. If you have to wait too long for an appointment, or if you don't have appropriate access to specialists, the quality of your care is negatively affected. Talk to a large number of people who are covered by managed care and you are going to hear a range of complaints about things such as the difficulty in getting answers to questions, denials of payment claims submitted, and waiting times for appointments. Sometimes people just

A NATIONAL RESEARCH CORPORATION SURVEY SHOWED THAT 66.1 PERCENT OF RESPONDENT RATED OVERALL QUALITY OF CARE AND SERVICE OF FEE-FOR- SERVICE PLANS AS EXCELLENT OR VERY GOOD COMPARED TO 60.2 PERCENT, FOR PPOS, AND 55.6 PERCENT FOR HMOS.

seem overwhelmed by what they see as the morass of managed care.

Some of these problems are caused by the members themselves. Often they have not read the policies and procedures of the plan, the "rules of the game," and since managed care is new to them they don't understand how it operates or how they should deal with this new form of health care.

Some of the complaints, such as denial of payment, are similar to those many people encountered under indemnity plans. Again, these are frequently a result of not understanding the rules.

All too often, however, the complaints are justified and are the result of poor performance on the part of the HMO.

HMOs are bureaucracies. Like other bureaucracies they need to constantly review their operations and their people. Good training is essential. But because of their rapid growth, many HMOs have not been able to keep up. Old management information systems (MIS) can't handle the load. New staff members are brought in without sufficient training, or the staffing is not adequate to the growing workload.

All of this gives managed care a bad name; perhaps not as bad as the horror stories reflect, but still bad. However, studies find the large majority of people are satisfied with their managed care plans.

A study by Care Data Reports showed that, overall, 60 percent of HMO members are satisfied with their plans. The ratings of specific plans in the study ranged from 45 percent up to 77 percent.

A recent study by CALPERS, the California Public Employees Retirement System, showed that 80 percent of members in HMOs were satisfied with their plan.

But in a survey of 170,000 U.S. households in 109 metropolitan areas conducted by the National Research Corporation, over 55 percent of respondents rated their plan as excellent or good. This compared unfavorably to a 66 percent rating for fee-for-service and a 60.2 percent rating for PPOs. A study published in the journal *Health Affairs* showed similar results with fee-for-service having a higher overall satisfaction than managed care.

CONSUMERS WHO HAVE A CHOICE TEND TO RATE THEIR HEALTH PLANS HIGHER.

A somewhat different picture resulted from a survey conducted by the Chicago Business Group on Health that found 84 percent of the 7,000 workers who responded were satisfied with their managed care plan.

Studies of managed care Medicaid and Medicare recipients demonstrated similar results. In Boston the satisfaction of Medicaid managed care recipients increased from 81 percent to 95 percent from 1994 to 1995.

A study by the federally sponsored Physicians Payment Review Commission found that 87 percent of Medicare recipients were satisfied with the care they received and did not face barriers to getting the care they needed.

While many people would still prefer the complete freedom of choice fee-for-service plans offer, the reality for most of us is to find a managed care plan that will satisfy us and meet our medical needs with quality care.

Despite the levels of satisfaction other people may enjoy in their HMO, if you have a problem the views of other members will not affect it.

There are many aspects of service, from the important issues mentioned above to more minor issues, such as long waits for appointments. Although the many aspects of service are difficult to enumerate, most people know what good service is even if they have no idea how to measure its quality. Once you're in a plan you can pretty easily judge the quality of service. The question is, how do you judge it before you're in the plan? Of course, one way is to ask as many people as possible who are in the plan (such as coworkers) about it, but since that is not always possible there are other ways you can assess the service component of a health plan.

Accreditation measures the quality of service to some degree, so it is likely an accredited HMO has met an acceptable standard of service quality. While accreditation is important, you can also use other means for making judgments about service quality.

Report Cards

Many HMO report cards describe ratings by members of various aspects of the HMO, including perceptions of quality and service. These satisfaction ratings are produced either by the HMOs themselves as they poll their members, or by employers or groups of employers who come together to assess the quality of health care they are paying for and their employees are receiving. An example of a report card is found below.

Aetna U.S. Healthcare® — Southeastern Pennsylvania
1996 HEDIS 3.0 Quality Report Card
Commercial HMO Population

Quality of Care Measure	Description	Rate
Member Access and Use of Services		
Adults' Access to Preventive Health Services	Adults who had an ambulatory visit in the past 3 years: • Age 20 to 44 • Age 45 to 64 • Age 65 and older	 82.4% 88.3% 91.6%
Well-Child Visits in the First 15 Months of Life	Children who had at least one well-child visit during the first 15 months of life	88.9%
Well-Child Visits in the Third through Sixth Year of Life	Children age 3 to 6 who had one or more well-child visits during 1996	70.9%
Adolescent Well-Care Visits	Adolescents age 12 to 21 who had one or more well-care visits during 1996	44.5%
Prevention and Screening		
Childhood Immunizations Mumps - Measles - Rubella (MMR) Diphtheria - Pertussis - Tetanus (DPT) Oral Polio Vaccine (OPV) Haemophilus Influenza, type B (Hib) Hepatitis B (HepB)	2-year-olds receiving the appropriate immunizations: • One MMR between ages 1 and 2 • Four DPTs by age 2 • Three OPVs by age 2 • One Hib between ages 1 and 2 • Two HepBs by age 2 • Overall immunization rate	 91.3% 84.6% 86.6% 84.3% 82.8% 68.3%

Adolescent Immunization Status	Adolescents who received a second dose of MMR by age 13	70.2%
Advising Smokers to Quit	Adults who received advice to quit smoking	69.9%
Breast Cancer Screening	Women age 52 to 69 who had a mammogram during the previous 2 years	78.1%
Cervical Cancer Screening	Women age 21 to 64 who had a Pap test during the previous 3 years	76.7%
Maternity Care		
Prenatal Care in the First Trimester	Women who received prenatal care in the first trimester	85.8%
Initiation of Prenatal Care	Women who had their first prenatal visit within six weeks of enrolling with the plan	
Check-ups After Delivery	Women who had a postpartum visit by the 42nd day after delivery	69.3%
Acute and Chronic Illness		
Treating Children's Ear Infections	Children who were prescribed a preferred antibiotic or no antibiotic for treatment of acute otitis media	56.9%
Beta Blocker Treatment after a Heart Attack	Adults who were prescribed a beta blocker after hospitalization for a heart attack	61.7%
Eye Exams for People with Diabetes	Diabetics age 31 and older who had an eye exam during 1996	39.8%
Follow-up after Hospitalization for Mental Illness	Ambulatory follow-up of patients hospitalized for treatment of a mental health disorder	77.9%
Member Satisfaction		
Overall satisfaction with the health plan	Responses of "completely satisfied," "very satisfied," and "somewhat satisfied"	80.7%
How has the plan's performance changed in the last 12 months?	Responses of "much better," "somewhat better," and "stayed the same"	92.9%
Would you recommend the health plan?	Responses of "definitely yes" and "probably yes"	87.7%

© Copyright 1997 U.S. Quality Algorithms®, Inc.

Some employers engage outside consultants to create report cards, while others manage the process through their own human resources departments. Usually only large employers have the resources to conduct such evaluations. However, these days smaller employers who come together in coalitions to purchase health insurance are also using their common interests to assess both quality of care and quality of service in the plans with which they contract. Often employers do not release their assessment to employees, instead using them to make management decisions about health plan purchasing.

You should check with your employer to see if report cards reflecting member ratings of service are available, either directly from the plans or from groups your employer may belong to that conduct assessments on the behalf of corporate members.

Governmental bodies and consumer groups also issue reports grading HMOs. The Center for the Study of Services, a non-profit organization, conducted a survey of HMOs that serve federal employees and released the results of those ratings. Some state governments also have conducted surveys of Medicaid recipients or of government employees. Appendix C contains summaries of consumer satisfaction surveys conducted by state health departments, consumer groups, large employers, the federal government, and consulting firms, as well as consumer groups that have conducted surveys of HMOs ratings by members. You may wish to contact these organizations for copies of these sur-

99 PERCENT OF HMOS AND 80.6 PERCENT OF PPOS CONDUCT CONSUMER SATISFACTION SURVEYS.

veys. However, since many of the HMOs assessed are regional or local, the results may not be fully applicable to plans in your community.

What follows is a list of possible questions for you to ask yourself — and any HMO you are considering — about various dimensions of service. Pose questions to the HMO service representative, or read the written material published by the HMO, to ascertain the answers. Permission is given to copy these pages and use them to make notes and a written record, so you will have them available for comparison.

Assessing Service:

What kind of informational material does the managed care plan distribute to members? Is it clearly written and does it contain good information? Does it answer your questions about the plan?

Can you join the plan if you are self-employed, or must you belong to a group? Must you undergo a physical examination first? If so, under what conditions can you be denied membership? Are there any conditions under which the plan can drop you from membership after you have joined?

Which hospitals are affiliated with the plan? Are you expected to use the emergency rooms of these hospitals in a crisis or is there a 24-hour emergency center? What happens if you go to another hospital?

What happens if you receive care outside of the plan's area? What documents must you submit and how long will you have to wait for reimbursement?

How do you leave the plan if you wish to? Do you have to wait a year to drop out? Will you be given your medical records if you leave, or can you arrange for them to be transferred to another doctor?

If you change health plans during the course of treatment, or while pregnant, can you stay with your current doctor until the treatment is completed?

Conversely, if your doctor leaves the plan, is he or she obligated to complete a course of treatment or will you need to find another doctor?

What are the procedures for staying with the plan if you leave your job but want to stay enrolled? Is that option available?

Does the plan have a full range of health promotion programs, such as nutrition, exercise classes and health education?

Does the managed care plan have central X-ray, laboratory, MRI, and pharmacy facilities? If not, where are these facilities located? Are they conveniently located with regard to your home or place of work?

How does one go about making an appointment?

How long do you have to wait to get an appointment for a checkup or for treatment of a specific problem? If you have an appointment, how long will you usually wait to see the doctor?

What are the procedures for referrals to specialists and subspecialists? Are there restrictions? What are they? Are the specialists you may need to see available to you?

What is the procedure for entering the hospital? Who do you have to notify, and when, on an emergency or non-emergency basis?

Assessing Service

Is there a formulary (list of approved drugs)?
Are generic substitutions made? Is it a formulary in
which substitutions can be made easily by participating doctors?

What is the procedure for seeking a
second opinion outside of the plan, if that is possible?

Is there a process for making an appeal if care has been denied,
such as tests, medical or surgical procedures, or second opinions?

How will any pre-existing conditions and illnesses
be handled, financially and medically?

What kind of grievance procedure does the plan have?

How many complaints were filed in the last year, and what were they about?
How were those complaints resolved?

In summary, you should expect good service from your managed care plan. You should not expect long waits for appointments. Your questions should be answered promptly, accurately and courteously. Paperwork should be processed in reasonable time. All the things you would expect as a special customer in any commercial enterprise should be reasonably expected. Why should good service in health care be the exception? Most importantly, your health care needs should be met.

You have to do your part, however. A simple thing like always carrying your membership card is important. Knowing the rules of the plan is also critical. Managed care plans, like other insurers, can act like mindless bureaucracies when you are "outside of the box." You need to work with the system and follow procedures and policies. If you do, things should work smoothly and effortlessly.

HMOs are well aware of the highly sensitive issue of service. Most work very hard to achieve high satisfaction levels because they are aware that it affects their reputation in the community. Some fall short of reasonable service, however, despite the efforts they may make.

How do you deal with a problem in service, or payments, or quality?

First, it is very important when dealing with any bureaucracy to keep accurate written records. When you first make a complaint, make a note of the date, time, to whom you spoke, and the result. If after two or three calls (all noted) your problem has not been resolved, put it in writing, including copies of any documentation, and cite your prior phone calls. Get the name of the appropriate person to write to, or at least the name and title of a senior officer, and address your letter to them. This usually gets a better response then a "Dear Sir or Madam" salutation. If you do not get a prompt response (and the definition of prompt can vary depending on the urgency of the issue) call the person's office. If you can't talk to them explain your problem to an assistant or secretary and request that someone call you back to discuss the issue. If you don't get a call back within 48 hours, pursue a formal grievance.

CALIFORNIA HAS THE HIGHEST PERCENT NATIONALLY OF MANAGED CARE — 38 PERCENT — AND ALASKA AND MISSISSIPPI THE LOWEST, WITH LESS THAN 1 PERCENT, ACCORDING TO DATA REPORTED IN *MODERN HEALTHCARE*.

Example of a letter you might send to an HMO, created by Michael H. Singer, an attorney specializing in health care law:

[Health plan name]
[Health plan address]
Attn: Directors of Appeals

Re: Appeal of Denial of [Benefits/Payments]
[Your Name]
[Case number (from their denial letter)]

Dear Sir or Madam:

I am writing you to formally appeal your health plan's decision to deny [necessary medical services/payment for necessary medical services]. I was informed of this denial by the enclosed "explanation of benefit" form, dated [insert date of form]. Your letter states that my [treatment/payment] is denied because of [insert reasons stated on form].

I disagree with your plan's denial of this claim, and believe that your decision denies me covered benefits. My reasons are as follows: [state the benefit that has been denied, and then refer to the page and paragraph of your employer's Summary Plan Description that describes the denied service as a covered benefit]. For your convenience, I am enclosing a copy of this page of the Summary Plan Description. [I am also enclosing a letter and supporting information from my plan physician that supports my claim.] I would appreciate receiving your decision as quickly as possible, and hope that I will hear from you within two weeks.

If you deny this appeal, please let me know the reasons why. It would be helpful for you to state the sections of my plan description that support your decision. Also, please include a list of all the medical records, x-rays, and reports that you reviewed in making this decision, and the specific portions that support your decision, so I can be sure that you have all of the available information and have not overlooked anything important. In addition, let me know the names of the people who made the decision and the name of a person I can contact to discuss your decision. Finally, please send a copy of your review/appeals procedures.

If you do not have complete medical information regarding this claim, or if you require any additional information, please let me know.

Sincerely,

[your name]
Attachments: Employer's Summary Plan Description (relevant pages only)
Copy of Plan's Denial Letter (Explanation of Benefits form)
Supporting letter and medical information from your plan physician

HMOs handle grievances in a variety of ways. However, their methods do share certain similarities. Grievances related to financial and administrative issues are typically reviewed by a committee made up primarily of the HMO's administrative staff. You begin the process by filing a formal complaint with the member services department following the procedures of the HMO.

If your complaint is denied some HMOs will permit a second review by a higher level committee. If you are still not satisfied you should write to the state agency that regulates HMOs in your state. It is usually the state insurance or health department.

Whatever route you take and whatever issue you are pursuing you should expect a timely resolution of your complaint. Of course, circumstances may influence the definition of timely.

Many health plans will respond to a grievance in 15 to 30 days. Some may take as long as 60 days to resolve an issue. When there are a number of appeals and denials, these issues can drag on for as long as six months.

In the case of denial of care for seriously ill patients, many HMOs have expedited procedures. In fact, the federal government mandates that seriously ill Medicare patients receive a response within 72 hours.

HMOs usually deal somewhat differently with issues

ONLY 50 PERCENT OF MARRIED CALIFORNIANS SURVEYED BY THE *LOS ANGELES TIMES* SAID THEY WERE IN THEIR HEALTH PLAN BECAUSE THEY PREFERRED IT. HOWEVER, 81 PERCENT RANKED THEIR PLANS AS GOOD OR EXCELLENT.

concerning denials or quality of medical care. They use what is termed the appeals process to handle these complaints. In this case the matter will be reviewed by a committee made up primarily of doctors and nurses. It is extremely helpful to have your doctor as an ally, supporting your case. If your doctor declines to do so, for whatever reason, seek a medical opinion outside of the plan and get it in writing. In cases concerning either denial or quality of care, the judgment of a physician is paramount. Also, if possible, get support from your employer. This can be especially helpful if your employer is a large one with many employees in a plan.

If your request is denied you may have the opportunity for another internal review by the HMO. Ultimately, as in the case of service issues, another level of appeal is to the appropriate state agency. Of course, it is also possible to take the matter to court, but that is a lengthy, time consuming and expensive process. In addition, many HMO contracts limit any appeal to the courts by requiring arbitration as a method of resolving these issues.

Consumers have not enjoyed much success in bringing HMOs to court, however. For many years managed care organizations have been shielded from malpractice suits, concerning denials or quality of care, by ERISA. Originally designed to protect retirement plans from suits, ERISA (the Employee Retirement Income Security Act of 1974) has been used successfully to protect health plans from malpractice suits.

Recently some courts have been punching holes in that

protective armor and refusing to let ERISA stand in the way of suits. A woman in Georgia, for example, recently won a $45 million dollar lawsuit against an HMO because it sent her sick child to a hospital 42 miles away where the HMO received discounts rather than to a nearby facility. On the way the baby went into cardiac arrest and sustained serious injuries. In another well-known case, a woman named Dukes successfully sued an HMO for punitive damages, claiming that the HMO's refusal to pay for a certain blood test that had been prescribed for her husband contributed to his death. The court found that the HMO could be held liable for punitive damages because its policies directly contributed to the patient's poor care. Many states are considering laws to remove the ERISA defense. The Texas legislature has passed a law designed to preempt ERISA and permit members to sue managed health care plans for poor treatment.

> **NINETY-ONE PERCENT OF HMO ENROLLMENT WAS IN MAJOR METROPOLITAN MARKETS IN 1995.**

Fortunately, most service problems can be resolved without resorting to state agencies or the courts. However, whether it is service, payment, denial of care or quality of care, you have to be assertive and well-prepared in pushing your case. Health plans are doing more and more to increase satisfaction rates, but sometimes the effective delivery of customer service falls behind ambitious goals. The quality of the service delivered can be strongly influenced by your willingness, and ability, to demand the best.

•Issues and Controversy•

Capitation

The practice of capitation, now common in HMO agreements with doctors, is at the heart of managed care philosophically, financially and operationally. It is a fundamental principle for putting the provider of care at risk for the cost of the care provided. Today, almost half of primary care services covered by HMOs are capitated.

The theory underlying capitation is the same one that applies to the HMO. Remember, an HMO is an insurance company. For a set, agreed upon fee, it guarantees to provide all necessary health care to its members. While few people have problems with this concept as applied to an insurance company, many resist the notion when it is applied to doctors, either individually or as a group.

As explained earlier, an HMO may contract with a network of doctors for the care of a large number of people. A group of 100 doctors in an IPA, for example, may agree to provide all of the primary care necessary for a population of 5,000 people. If the cost of the care exceeds the agreed upon amount — say $15 per month per patient — the doctors would lose money. Any money not spent on care would be profit to the network of doctors.

The logic behind capitation makes sense to its supporters, including many doctors. If doctors' decisions are behind 85 percent of health care expenditures, many argue that they should have the financial responsibility as well as the medical responsibility. Doctors will then be motivated to deliver cost-effective care and will do their utmost to keep patients healthy in order to reduce the need for expensive treatment options. It is the very logic behind the HMO!

Recently many critics of managed care, including some doctors, have rejected this logic. They suggest that doctors may have an incentive to deny required care if they, the doctors, could suffer financial losses.

On the other hand, many doctors want to accept capitation. It simplifies their billing and collecting and it gets all the non-medical managers, except those the doctors employ, out of the way. They see it as a way of returning authority for medical decision-making to doctors instead of leaving it in the hands of administrators.

Some studies have shown that when they are at risk for the cost of care, such as under capitation, doctors deliver care less expensively than when someone else is at risk.

Does this finding support the theory behind capitation and suggest that doctors can really find ways to deliver care more cost-effectively, or does it support what critics of capitation suggest, that doctors could be motivated to deny necessary care?

The answer to that question, of course, could be obtained from a comparison of the health status of patients cared for under a capitated system with the health status of patients cared for under another system. As of yet there is no definitive answer to this question. Most studies demonstrate no difference in the health status of people cared for by HMOs as compared to others. Many studies have concluded people in HMOs are as healthy as those insured in indemnity plans and use about the same amount of health care resources, with the exception of days spent in the hospital.

The widespread use of capitation is relatively new and critics contend that over time differences in health status will occur. As of yet, they have not, and it will take many more years and much more research to demonstrate differences if they exist. Since January 1, 1997, the federal government has required HMOs that participate in Medicare and Medicaid to reveal to the government, and to HMO members who ask, physician financial incentives.

You should discuss the issue of payment, and capitation in particular, with your doctor. How does your doctor view it and handle it? How will it affect your care? You need to build a trusting relationship with your doctor, whatever the compensation system. If you are not satisfied with the responses, you may have to consider changing doctors or plans — if that is possible.

Part Three

HOW TO MAKE THE BEST OF A MANAGED CARE PLAN

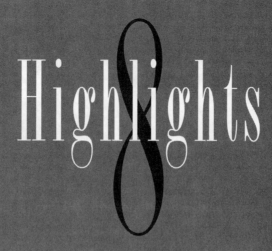

Highlights

Controlling costs is a priority in managed care. Some critics say HMOs manage costs, not care. This chapter reviews the various methods managed health plans use to control costs.

QUESTIONS ANSWERED IN THIS CHAPTER INCLUDE:

Has managed care controlled health care costs?

How do cost control efforts of HMOs affect physicians?

Is it true that clerks in HMOs review physicians orders?

Does my doctor need to get approval for everything she does to me?

Is it true that HMOs practice "cookie cutter" medicine?

How much do HMOs really focus on prevention?

Do HMOs restrict the drugs doctors can prescribe?

Controlling Costs

THE BOTTOM LINE
IS A TOP PRIORITY

This chapter is an in-depth examination of the way managed care controls costs. If you are not interested in this somewhat technical subject, feel free to skip ahead to chapter 9 (although the information in this chapter will help you to better understand managed care).

When the first staff and group HMO plans were established, such as Kaiser and HIP (Health Insurance Plan of New York), they controlled costs by having a central location, paying the doctors on salary, controlling all testing, and having well-developed utilization and care reviews. They held down costs primarily because they removed incentives for driving costs upward, which is an inherent part of indemnity insurance.

When the HMO concept began to boom in the eighties, many HMOs needed to do very little to really control costs. They could under-price indemnity plans simply by negotiating lower fees with doctors and hospitals, and cutting a little waste here and there. Many even lacked clinical information systems, and still were able to manage care well. However, as managed care enrollments grew and managed care penetration (the percent of people in a community insured through managed care plans) exceeded 40 percent, managed care plans found they were competing against each other and "managed indemnity" plans.

The result was that managed care plans not only had to focus on enrolling new members, but they also had to focus on the competition and *really* managing *costs*! In fact, this more aggressive focus on costs has led critics to suggest that managed care organizations manage costs, not care!

Learning how managed care health plans control costs is not only informative; an understanding of these techniques will help you get better care.

But be clear on one thing! Managed care has helped control health care costs. A few years ago there was some debate on this issue. Critics claimed that "cherry picking" was responsible. Today, there is virtually no debate.

One could cite a long list of studies demonstrating the impact of managed care on controlling health care costs, but a few examples may suffice.

Overall, health care costs in this country have slowed dramatically in the last few years and most experts attribute that to the influence of managed care. The increase in the Consumer Price Index (CPI) for health care has been reduced from 12.5 percent annually in 1981 to 3.9 percent in 1995. The average annual change in health benefit costs for active and retired employees has decreased from 18.6 percent in 1988 to a negative 1.1 percent in 1994.

A KPMG Peat Marwick LLP study, "The Impact of Managed Care in U.S. Markets," showed that hospital costs in high managed care markets were 11 percent below the national average and 19 percent below that of hospitals in low managed care markets.

A Hewitt Associates Health Value Initiative showed that HMOs were 18 percent more cost effective than indemnity plans.

A Millman & Robertson survey found that HMO rates declined for the second year in a row, by .07 percent, and that inpatient hospital days per 1,000 members decreased by 13.8 percent, from 275 in 1995 to 237 in 1996. An article in the *AMA News*, published by the American Medical Association, described price wars in the eastern part of the country among HMOs where rates were reduced 3-5 percent per year. And, of course, accompanying all of this, hospitals and doctors have seen their revenues — and hospitals their inpatient days — fall.

In Connecticut a committee of the state legislature concluded that HMOs in the state were reducing costs and satisfying consumers — something the legislature and public desired, one committee member suggested.

Towers Perrin, the benefits consulting firm, reported that in 1997 average monthly costs for indemnity coverage were $207 a month and coverage for HMOs and PPOs $196 and $157 a month respectively.

There is still debate surrounding the issue of whether or not managed care is saving the federal government

A JOHNSON AND HIGGINS SURVEY OF OVER 1,200 EMPLOYERS WITH FEWER THAN 1,000 EMPLOYEES SHOWED THEIR HEALTH COSTS ROSE ONLY 1.6 PERCENT IN 1995.

money on Medicare, but much of that debate centers on how the government is paying HMOs and how HMOs are selecting their new Medicare members (the cherry-picking issue) rather than on the effectiveness of managed care. Generally, the question being debated today is no longer *can* managed care control costs, but *how* it controls costs, and how these cost-saving techniques may affect quality.

The following pages will describe some of the methods managed care organizations use to control costs.

Cost-Saving Measures

Negotiating Fees

Because managed care organizations control the health care of so many people (large HMOs cover over a hundred thousand lives) they are able to negotiate discounts from doctors, hospitals, pharmacies, home care companies, and other providers. In exchange for the volume promised by managed care, providers are willing to discount prices. In fact, where managed care organizations enroll a large percentage of the population a provider has little choice but to participate. If 40 - 50 percent of the privately insured (not Medicare or Medicaid) people in a community are enrolled in managed care, and providers do not sign on and join a managed care network — or many networks — they could lose a substantial portion of their patients. For a doctor, hospital or other provider, that can be an impossible challenge. It is difficult to lose half of your patients and survive!

Changing Physician Incentives

In indemnity insurance programs, physicians are compensated for services they provide or procedures they perform. The more they do, the more they are paid. Many observers feel this is the primary financial reason why, under a purely indemnity insurance system, costs rose steadily from one year to the next.

Managed care organizations attempt to change this with a number of compensation arrangements. Some pay doctors a salary. Others discount traditional fee-for-service rates — only to find doctors increase the volume of services to compensate for the reduced rates. To control this, most health plans watch closely the tests and procedures doctors perform. Some health plans engage doctors in risk-sharing arrangements which provide that doctors gain if costs are controlled and suffer financially if budgets are exceeded.

Risk-Sharing

Risk-sharing can take a number of forms. One common risk-sharing mechanism is called a withhold or set-aside. As an example, a group of doctors may have a contract with an HMO to provide care to patients. A certain amount of their income or fees from the HMO, 20 percent for example, might be withheld or set-aside. If the group of doctors does not exceed budget for cer-

SEVENTY-SIX PERCENT OF STATE MEDICAID PROGRAMS NOW USE MANAGED CARE TO CONTROL COSTS, ACCORDING TO A STUDY BY INTEGRATED HEALTHCARE SERVICES.

tain services — the number of tests administered or referrals to other specialists — then they get to keep the 20 percent set-aside. If they exceed the budget they could lose some or all of the set-aside. This, of course, raises the issue of the doctor's motive in such cases; is it to save money and maintain the budget, or is it based on a medical judgment that found the test unnecessary? This kind of arrangement is not only troubling to doctors, but patients as well. In response to these concerns the federal government has required Medicare and Medicaid managed care plans to disclose physician pay arrangements that could compromise care. The legislation also requires physician groups to have stop loss insurance if they are at substantial risk, which is defined as withholds of more than 25 percent of total pay for a physician group that has fewer than 25,000 patients.

Another form of risk-sharing in wide use is capitation. Under capitation a group of doctors may receive a set dollar amount for the care of each person covered by a contract with an HMO. In some cases capitation may cover outpatient care; in other cases, it may include hospital care (inpatient), as well. The risk for the cost of care is carried by the doctor's group. If the costs exceed the amount budgeted they lose money. If the total costs are less than budgeted they make a profit. You should ask your doctor how he or she is compensated and discuss the impact of the system on your care.

Utilization Review

Among the methods initially used by managed care organizations to control costs are utilization reviews, pre-approvals, and case management. These techniques are used not only by managed care companies, but by almost all insurers these days. They are part of a continuing review of the care provided by a doctor, hospital, or other provider. They are unpopular with many doctors, who deeply resent their care of a patient being overseen or questioned by someone with less training than they have — a nurse, or even a clerical person using predetermined guidelines.

Retrospective utilization review is an after-the-fact review of a case. It attempts to determine if the care was appropriate and cost effective. Its primary goal is to be certain resources were not used wastefully.

Pre-Approval/Authorization

A doctor must receive prior authorization to perform a procedure or to hospitalize a patient. This rankles many doctors, but HMOs have found it an effective means of reducing hospitalization and reducing unnecessary procedures and tests.

Case Management and Continued Stay Reviews

A proactive form of management by an insurer, used most frequently in potentially complicated or expensive cases, case management involves a case manager,

SIXTY-NINE PERCENT OF HMOS PAY THEIR PRIMARY CARE DOCTORS ON A CAPITATED BASIS, ACCORDING TO INTERSTUDY.

usually a nurse, making certain the case is handled efficiently and appropriately. In its simplest form, it could entail ensuring that if a patient is to be admitted to a hospital for surgery, the appropriate tests are done in advance (hopefully, on an outpatient basis), that the surgery is scheduled promptly, that the patient is discharged as soon as possible, and that the follow-up care is appropriate. It can also verify that continued hospitalization is needed.

Practice Guidelines

Most patients don't realize it, but different doctors may treat the same problem by a wide variety of methods. For example, a recent major report, *The Dartmouth Atlas of Health Care*, concluded that in some communities radical mastectomies to treat breast cancer were performed at a rate 33 times as often as breast-saving lumpectomies. A man with early stage prostate cancer was four times as likely to have his prostate removed in Salt Lake City, Utah, than if he lived in Manhattan. A herniated disk was seven times more likely to be treated by surgery in a Tennessee community as compared to a community in Utah. In another study, one Connecticut community's rate of tonsillectomies was triple that of neighboring communities, with no difference in the health status of the children in those communities.

Other studies have demonstrated that the rate of hysterectomies performed on women in a community was more than double national averages — with no clear reason to justify the increased rate.

To address the issue of practice variations, many organizations such as the American College of Physicians, the Agency for Health Care Policy and Research, the American Medical Association and virtually all medical specialty groups, as well as many managed care organizations, have been active in developing clinical practice guidelines.

Managed care organizations have been among the leaders in this effort because they have the ability to know and to measure what hundreds of doctors are doing to thousands of patients. They also have direct and immediate access (if they have a good clinical management information system) to the records of all those patients. This is a wonderful resource for doing outcomes studies (i.e. studying the effectiveness of a treatment). In contrast, gathering the same information from hundreds of doctors who are not connected to each other in any way, who keep their clinical records in their own unique fashion, and who may have little incentive to participate in a time-consuming study, can be an extremely difficult challenge.

It is from this kind of patient database that clinical practice guidelines are developed. They describe what a group of experts has determined is the most effective way to treat a problem based on patient outcomes and cost. For example, is one drug more effective than another and at what cost? Once developed, they are shared with health care providers and, hopefully, widely used in treating patients. The result should be better

A STUDY BY KPMG PEAT MARWICK PUBLISHED IN *HEALTH AFFAIRS* DEMONSTRATED THAT COPAYMENTS FOR DOCTORS' VISITS IN HMOS TRIPLED FROM 1987 TO 1993, FROM AN AVERAGE OF $1.18 TO $4.15.

and more cost-effective care, an objective clearly in the interest of patients as well as managed care organizations. However, there is also some controversy surrounding practice guidelines, which some physicians label "cookie-cutter medicine." If you have a particular health problem, ask your doctor if there is a recommended practice guideline and if it is being followed. If not, why? And if variation from the guidelines is medically necessary, can the doctor do that without further authorization?

Prevention

Prevention is theoretically the heart of the Health Maintenance Organization. Of all the forms of managed care, HMOs stress prevention the most. The theory that by preventing illness you control costs is a sound one. Unfortunately, our nation, including the medical profession, has talked a good game of prevention but not put much real effort behind accomplishing it. Critics note that our entire health care system historically, with the exception of public health efforts such as providing potable water and sewage disposal, has been geared to illness, not wellness. Indemnity insurance usually has not reimbursed doctors for preventive care.

HMOs are supposed to emphasize preventive care. Some place strong emphasis on preventive services; some do not. Many HMOs issue report cards that show prospective enrollees and employers the degree of success they have achieved in delivering preventive care to their members. Preventive measures such as immunization of children, flu shots for adults, mammograms for women, and hypertension screening for those at risk, are routinely reported by HMOs. Also, the National Committee for Quality Assurance, the major accrediting organization for managed care, considers the delivery of preventive care as an important factor in its reviews.

While people enrolled in HMOs tend to receive more preventive services than others, many HMOs need to do much more. The preventive services described above are those focused on and measured. Since the results in delivering these services frequently become publicly available, HMOs are almost compelled to offer and even market them to members. However, while most HMOs offer these coverages, some do little to aggressively promote them to members. There are other preventive measures, such as preventive cardiac programs, that many HMOs do not even cover or, if they do, don't aggressively promote. The reason is that HMOs, like other insurers, realize that preventive care takes a long time to pay off and that many of the people they are serving today may be in a different program, managed care or indemnity, tomorrow. If a member is going to change plans, either because they change jobs or their employer contracts with a different insurer, or because the member wants to try a different plan, then why invest in expensive preventive measures that may not pay off for many years? It is a difficult economic argument to refute and large payers, government and employers, as well as individual consumers, need to demand that their HMOs deliver on

EIGHTY-ONE PERCENT OF MANAGED CARE ENROLLEES WERE REMINDED TO GET VACCINATIONS FOR THEIR CHILDREN, A RECENT STUDY BY CARE DATA REPORTED.

the promise of preventive care.

Demand Management

Many HMOs have initiated demand management programs which are often in the form of nurse information lines. These programs involve nurses available 24-hours a day to answer the questions and concerns of members. One important goal of such programs is to reduce costs by avoiding unnecessary visits to the emergency room or to doctors. The nurses can provide a great deal of basic health information as well as outline options for responding to various symptoms. The nurses do not provide care but information, and they are guided by well-developed protocols in responding to problems.

Disease State Management

A more sophisticated form of prevention being employed by an increasing number of HMOs is called disease state management. Recognizing that many people with chronic illness, such as diabetes or hypertension, end up being very expensive patients because some of them let their disease get out of control, HMOs are creating or contracting out special programs to closely manage members with these diseases. By developing some clinical practice guidelines and managing the disease states through these guidelines, HMOs find that they can prevent more serious problems requiring intensive (and expensive) care or often hospitalization, from developing. Such an approach is good for patients as well as for the bottom line! At the same time, an HMO may try not to become too well known for such programs out of fear that people with chronic diseases may flock to it, thus driving up costs. An entire new industry is being created these days by companies offering demand management and disease state management programs to HMOs, employers, and others. From companies with nurses and doctors on call, to companies that manage specific diseases like heart disease, cancer, and diabetes, frequently assuming the risks of total care for these patients (often called disease state carve-outs), there is a new emphasis on reducing expensive care through better management of chronic disease. When you realize that about 69 percent of hospital admissions, 80 percent of bed days and 96 percent of home care visits are generated by patients with chronic illnesses, you can appreciate the scope of the problem and the potential for savings.

ALMOST ONE-HALF OF ALL MANAGED CARE PLANS HAVE CLOSED FORMULARIES.

Formularies

HMOs generally present members with a list of drugs that are approved for coverage and, therefore, for use by patients. These lists are called formularies. Open formularies, used by about 30 percent of HMOs, are lists of suggested drugs; physicians are not required to stick to the list. Closed or restricted formularies, used by approximately 68 percent of HMOs, are more restrictive, and a physician may have to seek approval to prescribe a drug not on the list. Whenever possible, most HMOs use generic rather than brand name drugs to save money, and generics make up a large part of for-mulary lists. Occasionally this becomes an issue when a doctor wants to prescribe, or a patient requests, a drug not included in the formulary because the gener-ic drug does not work the same for this particular patient as the branded drug. This is not a common issue because generic drugs are approved by the FDA (Food and Drug Administration) of the federal govern-ment only after they have been proven to be safe and biologically equivalent to the brand-name drug. However, on occasion there are individuals who react differently to a brand-name drug and its generic coun-terpart. In such cases doctors and patients need to appeal to use the branded product. There is a signifi-cant debate about the effectiveness of formularies these days. Some people believe they may cost more than they save and there is some discussion about HMOs moving away from formularies, but most HMOs still have them. If you are joining an HMO and use a par-ticular medication, check to see if it is part of the for-mulary and, if not, how you might continue using it.

Buying Power

Like other large organizations, managed care organiza-tions use their size and buying power to buy things less expensively. As a result, enrollees covered by managed care are often able to enjoy broader benefits (coverages) than people insured by indemnity plans. Drug purchas-ing plans, for example, are a common benefit in man-aged care. Many HMOs offer prescription drug plans.

Pharmacies frequently complain about this kind of "market muscle" and many small, local pharmacies who have difficulty becoming part of managed care networks are facing a tremendous challenge, but the managed care member benefits by lower prices and expanded benefits.

Buying power was the first and greatest leverage managed care brought to the health care competitive market. Many managed care organizations initially did little to manage care. With their buying power, they negotiated discounts with doctors, hospitals and other providers — say a 20 percent discount — and then priced their coverage 10 percent below indemnity insurance (called "shadow pricing"), making a profit. However, intense competition has led managed care organizations to actively apply all of these cost control measures to the delivery of care in order to compete not only with indemnity insurance, but with each other.

While both patients and providers may complain at times about one or all of these measures, there is a general recognition that managed care has been the primary force behind slowing the growth of health care costs. Many critics of managed care seem to have forgotten that it was only a few years ago, in the early nineties, that the substantial increases in health care costs were threatening our entire system of financing care. Between 1960 and 1990 health care spending grew at a rate of 6 percent annually after adjustments for inflation. This was more than double the growth rate of any

OVER 50 PERCENT OF HMOS SURVEYED BY INTERSTUDY IMPLEMENTED DISEASE MANAGEMENT PROGRAMS. ASTHMA WAS THE PRIMARY AREA OF FOCUS, FOLLOWED BY DIABETES (45.5 PERCENT).

EMPLOYERS

WITH 500 OR

MORE EMPLOY-

EES SPEND

ABOUT $1.60 FOR

EACH HOUR

WORKED ON

HEALTH CARE

COSTS. SMALL

EMPLOYERS,

1-99 EMPLOYEES,

SPEND ABOUT

$.80 PER HOUR

WORKED.

other area of spending. Indemnity insurance coverage in some communities reached an annual cost of $12,000 per family! Private employers and government payers were rebelling, small employers were dropping health care insurance from their benefit plans, and proposals were being made for a government takeover of health care. The debate has now shifted from controlling costs to doing so while providing quality.

The key for you, as a consumer and patient, is to make certain that these cost saving measures improve the quality of your care, and do not harm it. Before you join a health plan, ask a service representative about wellness and preventive care programs available to members. Ask for report cards. And if you have a chronic disease, ask about the clinical protocols the plan uses. Also ask if they have special programs — "centers of excellence" — to treat people with that problem.

•Issues and Controversy•

Provider Selection

Earlier we explored the issue of "cherry-picking," a process whereby health insurers, both indemnity and managed care, are accused of selecting young, healthy people as members whenever possible. While that issue has diminished in recent years, another issue has gathered steam — provider selection. HMOs need to control both costs and quality. Part of that control comes from selecting doctors who meet their criteria, accept their fees or other compensation arrangements, and follow their policies. Initially, many doctors resisted managed care. Why accept lower fees and have some organization tell you how to practice medicine? But as HMOs enrolled more and more people, doctors had little choice but to participate.

Some doctors held out too long and when they wanted to join a managed care network, it was too late. They weren't needed! The result was many lost a large portion of their patient base, a severe financial hardship.

Other doctors are excluded because they do not meet the criteria mandated by managed care organizations. Doctors who are not board certified, for example, are often excluded. This credentialing process is something that indemnity insurers do not do. They do not screen providers in any way, except to be sure they have a billing number. Most HMOs not only screen providers based on quality prior to admitting them to their networks, but also review them on an ongoing basis.

Because this is such an important issue to both doctors and HMOs, it has ended up in the courts and in many state legislatures under the label of "any willing provider." Doctors' groups are suing HMOs, or advocating legislation to require HMOs to include in their network any doctor who is willing to accept the fees and follow the policies of the HMOs.

The HMOs respond that they cannot control costs and quality and have a well-functioning, efficient, network if they are not free to be selective in organizing their networks. They argue, correctly, that if they cannot promise volume to their doctors, they cannot negotiate discounts. This issue is currently being fought in a number of courts and legislatures around the country. The most significant impact on a consumer occurs when your doctor cannot join the plan to which you belong. At times, doctors have followed patients into HMOs. For example, in a community where many of the adults are employed by one large employer and a doctor's practice is comprised primarily of this group, being part of an HMO that covers these people can be critical. For the most part, however, this is a struggle between HMOs and doctors and does not directly impact patients unless your doctor is excluded from a plan you must join.

Selection of providers is a critical issue to more than doctors. Hospitals, pharmacies, chiropractors, physical therapists and practitioners of alternative therapies are all concerned about being excluded from managed care networks. Again, it is a competitive market issue. If you are not part of a network that enrolls thousands of people in your service area, you cannot provide care to them. If you are not part of some networks, and managed care dominates health care in your community, you could be out of business!

In the early days of managed care, some hospitals resisted the discounted rates offered by HMOs. Today they aggressively compete to be part of managed care networks. In many cases it is a matter of survival.

The same is true for many of the other providers mentioned. In some states, chiropractors are trying to get legislatures to pass regulations requiring that HMOs cover chiropractic care.

Local pharmacies that are not part of large chains have had difficulty becoming part of managed care. An HMO would rather negotiate one contract that covers 100 pharmacies than negotiate with 100 individual pharmacies. As a result, pharmacies and other individual providers, including individual doctors, are organizing into groups to negotiate with managed care organizations. Willing provider legislation is being called for by many of these providers who are concerned about their survival.

Managed care organizations are consolidating and merging. This stimulates consolidation of the providers that serve them. The result of these vast market changes is larger organizations with greater negotiating power and fewer "stand-alone" providers. These changes are the most rapid and dramatic forces that have affected health care in decades.

Becoming affiliated with a managed care network is important for doctors and other providers, but staying affiliated is also important.

Doctors have accused some HMOs of dropping them unfairly because of the high cost of the care their patients required. This is of particular concern to those doctors who have many older or chronically ill patients. The HMOs have denied these charges and said there were other reasons for dropping the doctors, such as quality.

The doctors who have made these charges claim the HMOs are using "economic credentialing," judging the doctor's performance not on the quality of care, but on the cost of the care the doctor delivers.

It is a difficult issue to sort out. It is estimated that decision making by doctors controls or influences 85 percent of health care expenditures. Clearly, HMOs want doctors who follow their policies and guidelines — if they do not have a negative impact on patient care. If the policies do interfere with patient care, we all want a doctor who will be a strong patient advocate.

If a single doctor in a community complains about an HMO practicing economic credentialing, it should not be of great concern to patients because it could be an individual matter. However, if a number of doctors begin publicly complaining about being dropped from an HMO because they provided "too much" care, there may be a real issue to which HMO members should be sensitive. Most doctors do not seek public controversy, and if an issue like economic credentialing becomes public, consumers should be watchful.

The most recent trend that has emerged is the formation of Physician Practice Management companies (PPMs). These companies organize large networks of doctors, often actually buying their practices, with the goal of negotiating with Managed Care Organizations (MCOs) and, in many cases, providing cost efficiencies and improved practice management to the physician groups.

Notes & Phone Numbers

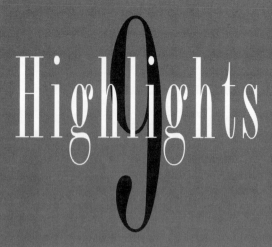

Highlights

While your insurance plan is important, your doctor is even more important in making certain you get the best care possible. Selecting the right doctor is as critical as selecting the right plan.

QUESTIONS ANSWERED IN THIS CHAPTER INCLUDE:

My health plan requires I choose a primary care physician. What kind of doctor should I select?

What does it mean if a doctor says he is board certified?

How can I check on a doctor's credentials and certification?

The Doctor of Choice

YOUR PRIMARY CARE PHYSICIAN

If you have recently received an introductory package from a new HMO you know the scenario: You open the thick book of participating physicians and quickly scan the pages to find the name of your own physician. If the name is there, you breathe a sigh of relief. If the familiar name does not appear, you throw up your hands in resignation and simply choose a doctor the way you might select a hardware store — one that is close to home, knowing little about the doctor's qualifications or professional practice set-up. If the momentous event of choosing a primary care doctor still remains in your health care future, you need to know how to choose the best. Even if you have already made a choice, you need to know if it was the right one. If your doctor is part of your new health plan, don't assume that it will be "business as usual." Your future relationship with your current doctor could be changed in many ways.

A very positive requirement of virtually all HMOs is that you choose a primary care physician (the shortened term these days is PCP). This doctor becomes the "quarterback" of your medical team, guiding you through the sometimes challenging playing field of our health care system. Often referred to as a "Gatekeeper," the primary care physician also controls your access to the other resources of the HMO, such as tests, procedures and other specialists. Virtually nothing happens to you in an HMO unless your primary care doctor approves it, although, as will be described in Chapter 10, that may be changing.

Mandating that members have a primary care doctor is one of the strongest aspects of HMOs. Too many Americans get poor health care at excessive cost by bouncing from specialist to specialist without anyone really being "their doctor." Another value of HMOs is that they usually review the credentials of their doctors very carefully, which is something indemnity insurers do not do.

Here are the four most important criteria upon which you should base your selection of a primary care physician. Your HMO should have all the necessary information available and provide it upon request.

One: Specialty

Selecting the right kind of doctor as a primary care physician is relatively easy since the choices are limited to four. For a child, there is the possibility of a pediatrician or a family practitioner. For an adult male the choice could be a family practitioner or an internist. For an adult female, an obstetrician/gynecologist, family practitioner, or internist are possible choices. There are no clear rules for guiding your choices. It is a matter of preference.

Family practitioners care for both adults and children. In some states they may deliver babies and perform or assist in surgery. They fit the old concept of the "family doctor." They are found in greater numbers in the South and Midwest and in many rural communities. They are a smaller proportion of the medical practitioners in major cities, especially in the northeast.

Internists care for adults, not children. They are trained to handle all aspects of internal medicine. If you have a chronic disease, such as cardiac disease, you may want to find an internist who is also board certified in cardiology. These days, because of the demand for primary care specialists, many internists who have subspecialty training practice a mix of their subspecialty and primary care. Many of these physicians choose to focus in a subspecialty area such as cardiology, gastroenterology, or geriatrics.

Obstetrician/Gynecologists are not trained to be primary care physicians, according to the American Academy of Obstetrics and Gynecology, but the reality is that many women use their gynecologist for primary care. A study by the American Academy of Obstetrics and Gynecology demonstrated that about 54 percent of women use their Ob/Gyn for primary care. Your HMO may or may not consider Ob/Gyn specialists as primary care physicians.

Pediatricians are the medical specialists most commonly used for the care of children and adolescents. In fact, adolescent medicine is a new subspecialty of both Pediatrics and Internal Medicine. These doctors are an appropriate choice for a child's primary care physician.

OVER 81 PERCENT OF HEALTH PLANS THAT RESPONDED TO AN AAHP/KAISER FAMILY FOUNDATION SURVEY PERMITTED MEMBERS TO SELECT AN OB/GYN AS A PRIMARY CARE PHYSICIAN OR SELF-REFER TO ONE. ABOUT 20 PERCENT REQUIRED A NEW REFERRAL FOR EACH OB/GYN VISIT.

Some HMOs have been experimenting with Licensed Nurse Practitioners as primary care providers. As a patient you should have the right to choose the kind of health care professional you want to care for you. If you prefer a Licensed Nurse Practitioner, fine; if not, then request a primary care physician.

Two: Board Certification

This qualification is not just a nice added extra, it is virtually imperative. A board certified physician has completed an approved residency program and passed a rigorous exam in a recognized medical specialty such as internal medicine, surgery, psychiatry, pediatrics or dermatology.

If a physician is not board certified you have no assurance of specialized training. In fact, in some states anyone who has completed medical school and only one year of residency can "hang out a shingle" as a surgeon, a urologist, a gynecologist or practice in any medical specialty!

While board certification does not guarantee the doctor is excellent, or even good, at least you are assured of appropriate training. "Board eligible" is a term some physicians use to describe themselves, but it has no official meaning in the view of the American Board of Medical Specialties (ABMS). It does mean that the doctor has completed a residency and is eligible to take the board exam. It can also mean the doctor took the exam twice and failed and does not plan to take it again, thus remaining "board eligible." With younger physicians, it may be an accurate description of their status, but with older physicians it has less meaning.

If a physician is not board certified, you need to be assured they have at least completed a residency in their specialty (ask them) and/or have years of practical experience and an excellent reputation in their community, among practitioners as well as the public. Nurses and other health professionals are often good "reference checks."

All of the specialty medical boards require doctors to be recertified as well. Certification periods may last from eight to ten years and the doctors take a recertification exam as well as demonstrate that they have completed continuing medical education (CME) courses. Recertification ensures your doctor is making an effort to keep up with changes in the field.

There are a number of ways to check on a physician's board certification. The American Board of Medical Specialties publishes the *Directory of Medical Specialists* which is available in most libraries. You can also call the ABMS at (800) 776-2378 to ask about a physician's certification status. In addition the American Medical Association (AMA) has a web site (http://www.ama-assn.org) where you can check on a physician's education and training, including board certification. Often hospitals, state and county medical societies, or the doctor's office will provide the information.

A KAISER FAMILY FOUNDATION SURVEY SHOWED THAT MORE THAN THREE-QUARTERS OF THE PEOPLE SURVEYED SAID THEY WOULD PICK A DOCTOR THEY KNEW OVER ONE THEY DID NOT KNOW — EVEN IF THE STRANGER HAD MUCH HIGHER QUALITY RATINGS.

Three: Hospital Affiliation

Another important consideration in selecting a primary care physician is the doctor's hospital appointment. If you need to be hospitalized, it is very likely that you will be admitted to the hospital where your primary care physician is on staff.

The best hospitals attract the best doctors, and since hospital care is usually a team effort, you want the best team possible. Managed care organizations typically contract with a number of hospitals. This is especially true of large plans. Try to find a doctor on the staff of one of the best hospitals in the MCO network when you are choosing your primary care physician.

One important note: If you see the names of several excellent hospitals, ask the MCO service representative what kind of contract they have with the managed care organization. Frequently MCOs contract with some hospitals only for specific services (e.g. cardiac surgery, oncology) and other hospitals for general care. Don't assume a hospital you see listed, even if close to where you live, is accessible for all purposes.

Four: Compatibility

The chemistry between you and your doctor is also an important consideration in your choice of a primary care physician. The doctor's personality and manner of interacting with patients, which we often refer to as "bedside manner," will significantly affect the chemistry between you and your physician. Patients want doctors who listen to them and demonstrate concern about their health.

Chemistry is critical. You need to have a doctor you respect and trust and whom you feel respects you as a patient. During your first appointment with your primary care doctor — which you should schedule immediately upon joining a plan — you should assess this issue of the chemistry between you carefully. Some points to consider are:

Involving Patients in Decision Making – Some patients simply accept whatever a doctor tells them; others want to be involved in making decisions about their medical care. Some doctors deliver care in an authoritarian manner; others are more open to discussing issues and questions with their patients. This is one of the things you and your doctor need to agree upon and be comfortable with in your interaction. Discuss it openly with your doctor.

Practice Arrangements – Is the doctor in solo practice or in a group? Who covers for the doctor when he or she is not available? Will the doctor accept phone calls from patients? Visit patients in their homes?

Ethical and Religious Issues – These issues are often extremely important to people. They are sensitive and serious issues. Discuss them with a physician you are considering as your primary care provider.

SIXTY-FOUR PERCENT OF THOSE SURVEYED BY CARE DATA IN A STUDY OF HMO MEMBERS WERE PLEASED WITH THEIR PRIMARY CARE PHYSICIANS.

Changing Your Physician

There are times, whether you are in managed care or covered by indemnity insurance, that you should change your physician. In managed care settings, however, this option may be limited by the policies of the HMO. You may be able to change primary care providers only once or twice a year. This should not be a problem. If you do a little research beforehand and select your doctors carefully, changes should be infrequent.

Some of the reasons that may prompt you to consider changing include:

Poor bedside manner

Vague and evasive answers to questions

Never on schedule

Cannot diagnose a problem

Discourages second opinions

Unpleasant office staff

Violates medical privacy

Whenever you consider leaving a doctor you should discuss the reasons. You should also make certain you have copies of all your medical records; whether you are in managed care, or covered by indemnity insurance, this is a good practice and, in most states, your legal right. Having your medical records can help a new doctor better understand your health history and status, and it may save repeating tests and, as a result, money!

Choosing a Primary Care Physician

Is the doctor thorough in his/her exam?

Does he or she listen to you carefully? Answer your questions?

Does the doctor explain things carefully in understandable terms?

Are you comfortable with the doctor's views on the use of medications, tests, important ethical issues?

Did you feel rushed?

Were you able to get a prompt call back when you called the doctor's office?

Does the doctor have adequate coverage for times when he or she is on vacation or otherwise unavailable?

Did the doctor's staff treat you courteously?

•Issues and Controversy•

Referrals to Specialists

One of the very sound and fundamental principles of managed care is the reliance on primary care physicians to deliver preventive and basic medical care, and to appropriately utilize referrals to other specialists. It is for this reason that primary care doctors are often referred to as "gatekeepers," a label many resist .

Patients in some HMOs have complained that their primary care doctors have been too slow to refer them to other specialists, when they, the patient, felt they needed the care of another specialist or subspecialist. This issue has been a major point of contention between HMOs and their members. In fact, it has prompted some HMOs to permit patients to see specialists without a referral from a primary care physician. Sometimes these plans are described as "non-gatekeeper" or "HMOs without walls." Their goal is to remove what some consumers believe to be restraints on choice.

The media coverage of the issue of referrals to specialists has been negative for HMOs. A California HMO was fined $500,000 by the state for failing to make medically necessary referrals. The case involved a nine-year-old girl with a rare tumor who was denied access to a specialist with extensive experience in her problem. Fortunately, the surgeon operated, but when the HMO refused to pay not only his bill but the hospital's bill, even though the hospital was part of its network, the child's parents sued.

Some doctors also have expressed concern about this issue, but from a somewhat different perspective. The concern of the doctors, primarily subspecialists, is that primary care doctors are sometimes reluctant to refer patients because they may incur some financial penalty and are instead treating the patients themselves. These specialists complain that not only are the primary care doctors depriving them of income, but they are often offering care or performing techniques for which they are not properly trained.

When you believe you need the care of a specialist, discuss it with your primary care doctor. If he or she will not refer you, and the conversation has not changed your mind, appeal to the medical director of the HMO. If all else fails you may want to pay for a visit to a specialist yourself. If you believe the problem to be serious, it may be worth it! Also, when being referred to a specialist make certain that the physician has the appropriate training and expertise to deal with your problem. If not, appeal to the HMO and, if necessary, demand to be referred to someone who can deal with the problem appropriately.

Highlights

10

How you interact and relate to your doctor is as important as selecting the right doctor. Managed health plans may have an impact on your relationship with your doctor.

QUESTIONS ANSWERED IN THIS CHAPTER INCLUDE:

How do HMOs limit my choice of doctors?

Is getting referrals to a specialist a major problem?

How do I get to see a specialist if I need one?

Does managed care affect the way my doctor practices medicine?

Can I still trust my doctor, or are HMO rules and money in the way?

Is it true that the best doctors don't join HMOs?

You and Your Doctor

A CRITICAL RELATIONSHIP

The area where a managed care plan can affect you most greatly is your relationship with your doctor. It is both the perceived impact and the real impact to which you and your doctor must adapt.

In the best of circumstances, the corporate HMO will completely fade into the background of your relationship with your doctor. Some people join an insurance plan because they know their doctor is in it and, consequently, never feel intruded upon as members of an HMO or part of managed care. This kind of experience is not typical, however.

Making Choices in a Different Way

The first, and perhaps most important way managed care affects you and your doctor is on the matter of choice. Your selection of doctors, both for primary care and for other specialists, is limited. One way some people characterize managed care is to describe it as a trade-off of choice for reduced costs, expanded coverages and less paperwork. Whatever your view of it, positive or negative, the issue is simple: One of the underlying principles of managed care is limiting patient choice to those doctors, hospitals and other providers who have chosen and been allowed to participate in the plan; who agree to follow its procedures; and who agree to accept its fees and thus become part of the plan's network.

Managed care organizations claim they must do this to control costs and quality. They state they need to select quality doctors who deliver cost-effective patient care according to the standards and procedures of the managed care plan. In fact, many HMOs require board certification as a minimum qualification, and this, as well as other issues involved in selecting doctors to be part of networks, has created controversy with doctors in some communities.

The issue of choice is a real one. About 40 percent of people who join HMOs have to change their primary care doctor. Unfortunately, if your employer changes plans or your doctor leaves the plan you will have to choose a new doctor. Americans feel strongly about wanting to choose the doctors and hospitals that will care for them. To overcome the issue of lack of choice, many managed care plans have responded by creating the Point of Service plan (POS) to give members freedom of choice of doctors and hospitals at additional cost to the member.

Referrals to Specialists

Managed care also limits your choice of specialists and subspecialists. In most cases you will not be able to see another specialist without a referral from your primary care doctor, and you will be limited to the specialists in the network unless your injury or illness is so complex and so highly specialized that the HMO will authorize referrals to specialists not in their network. Referral to specialists outside of a network is an issue of concern to many people. Some cases where HMOs have refused to let people be cared for by specialists out of the network, when the patient felt doctors within a network were not the best to care for a particular problem, have drawn national attention. While such cases are rare, they vividly demonstrate the conflict between choice on one hand and controlling costs on the other.

Managed care organizations have to control access to specialists in order to control costs. A managed care plan cannot afford to have members unilaterally deciding when and why they need to see an orthopedist, an endocrinologist, a rheumatologist, or any of the other various medical specialists and subspecialists and, at the same time, continue to control costs or quality.

Referrals are one of the trickiest issues in managed care. Traditionally, doctors developed their own referral networks. They may have referred to doctors in their own medical group, if it was a multi-speciality practice, or there may have been doctors on the same hospital staff to whom they referred.

Managed care can dramatically change the normal referral patterns. MCOs negotiate agreements with various kinds of specialists, either individuals or groups,

A STUDY IN *HEALTH AFFAIRS* SHOWED THAT PEOPLE ENROLLED IN HMOS AND PPOS VISITED THEIR DOCTORS MORE THAN PEOPLE COVERED BY INDEMNITY INSURANCE (4.8, 4.5 AND 4.0 ANNUAL VISITS RESPECTIVELY).

for specific services. For example, a MCO may negotiate with a large group of ophthalmologists to provide eye care to its members, or with a hospital and a group of cardiac surgeons for all of its open-heart surgery. One unfortunate result is that sometimes primary care doctors end up making referrals to doctors who are in the network, but they don't know on a personal or professional basis. But if a group of physicians has the contract for those services, there is no alternative.

Whatever the arrangement, you can be sure that in most cases the MCO has a limited number of specialists under contract for specialized care and that your choice, unless you are in a Point of Service plan (POS), will be restricted to those doctors. You should be certain there is an adequate number of each kind of specialist in the plans you are considering.

Despite these arrangements, for the most part you will have choices in specialty services through your primary care physician. Few HMOs have only one doctor providing a certain kind of care. Even in small HMOs you will usually have a choice of a number of physicians. When your primary care doctor suggests someone for a referral you should ask a few basic questions of your primary care doctor.

Referrals to Specialists

Why is your doctor recommending this particular doctor?

With what hospitals is the doctor affiliated?

Could your primary care doctor suggest two or three specialists rather than one?

If you are being referred for a particular procedure,
what is the doctor's experience with that procedure?

If you are not satisfied with the answers, ask for some other options. Referring you to a doctor simply because "that's what the plan calls for" is not good enough. When you have a particularly difficult or complex problem, you want to be certain the physician to whom you are referred is certified in the appropriate subspecialty and has had training and experience with the problem. For example, if you have a problem with your endocrine system you want to be certain you will be treated by a board certified endocrinologist. If you need surgery on your wrist or hand, you want to be operated on by a board certified hand surgeon.

You should ask your primary care physician and, if he or she doesn't have the information, the medical director of the HMO about the qualifications of doctors to whom you are being referred.

Of course, you will want to do your own checking on

the doctor to whom you are referred, e.g. board certification, fellowship training, etc. Also, once you see the specialist be certain to tell your primary care physician your assessment of your care, positive or negative.

Second opinions should be handled in similar fashion. If you feel a second opinion is warranted, ask for it. You may want to do this if your physician's diagnosis seems uncertain, turns out not to be correct, or you have received different assessments over time or from different doctors. You may feel more comfortable going outside the network for a second opinion. In any case, you want to be certain the physician is well trained and experienced in dealing with your problem.

If your options are truly limited and you don't feel the doctor and/or the hospital to which you are being referred, either for care or for a second opinion, is of satisfactory quality, appeal to your primary care doctor and, if necessary, to the plan for other options. Even if you have to go outside the network and pay more, it's worth it to obtain quality. But be judicious in your use of expensive medical resources. Many people, especially under indemnity insurance, get poor care from excellent doctors because they bounce from doctor to doctor and no one physician ever knows them well enough to provide good quality care. Remember, poor quality health care is the most expensive health care and it also can be the most risky!

If you do violate the policy of the HMO and see a specialist without a referral from your primary care doctor,

> A STUDY BY THE NATIONAL RESEARCH CORPORATION SHOWED THAT 22.9 PERCENT OF HMO ENROLLEES WERE NOT ABLE TO GET REFERRALS TO SPECIALISTS, AS COMPARED TO 6.1 PERCENT IN FEE-FOR-SERVICE PLANS.

you undoubtedly will pay for it — unless you are in a POS plan that permits it. Even then you will be required to pay at least 20 - 30 percent of the physician's fee, and if you haven't followed the procedures for going outside of the network, you may pay all of it!

Due to the strong desire for choice on the part of American consumers, Point of Service Plans (POS) are a fast growing option in managed care and, in fact, some HMOs are initiating "managed care without walls," permitting members to see specialists without a referral from a primary care physician.

Reviews and Authorizations

While you will be limited in your choice of doctors, your doctor's choice of how to care for you will be limited by HMO policies. Where you are hospitalized for particular procedures or services will be restricted to plan hospitals. The drugs your doctor prescribes, and the other physicians you may be referred to, will all be guided by HMO policies. Even the way in which your doctor cares for you may be guided by HMO approved protocols.

All of this is a part of controlling costs, but none of it should affect the quality of your care. The resources your doctor can use to care for you should be of high quality; if not, your doctor would not be part of the plan. Many of these policies, such as using well-tested and practiced protocols, should improve your care.

However, the reality is that your doctor's care will be provided within the policies of the health plan you join. This is why it is so important to select the best health plan possible.

Paying for Care

Making Payments in a Different Way

COSTS OF OUTPATIENT CARE ARE CUT IN HALF WHEN PATIENTS VISIT A PRIMARY CARE PHYSICIAN FIRST, ACCORDING TO A STUDY CONDUCTED BY JOHNS HOPKINS SCHOOL OF PUBLIC HEALTH.

One positive way managed care affects the relationship between you and your doctor is by getting issues about fees and billing out of the examining room. Typically, you and your doctor will not have to deal with this issue. The doctor will have agreed in advance with the managed care plan on compensation and, if you need to pay anything, such as a small copay, you will usually pay at the doctor's office.

Billing procedures are a minor issue, but they raise another very significant point: doctor compensation. Many people, including patients, are concerned about a compensation system within which, in effect, rewards are offered for not delivering care. The concern is that some doctors may be reluctant to administer even necessary care in cases where the bottom line may be called into question. The compensation arrangements used by managed care, including capitation and set-asides, can raise troubling ethical issues for doctors and patients. Fortunately, the overwhelming motivation for most doctors is to do what is best for their patients. They have committed their lives to that principle.

Nonetheless, it would be foolish to ignore the reality that financial incentives affect the behavior of all people, including doctors. Discuss compensation issues with your doctor if you believe they could affect your care.

Trust: The Lost Connection

You need to have confidence in your doctor, because your primary care physician should be your advocate in the managed care setting. While the initial responsibility for getting the best care is yours, you need to trust that your doctor, despite any uncertainties in the system, is going to be your advocate and ensure that you are getting what you need as a patient over the long term.

You should ask your doctor about the HMO's method of compensation. Is it a capitation system? Are there set-asides? Is there anything in the arrangement with the managed care organization that would negatively influence your doctor's care for you? If there is, you and your doctor need to discuss it. You have to make certain you are comfortable with the arrangement and trust the doctor in any and all circumstances. If you don't feel that trust, you may need to change doctors or plans, although these days finding a managed care plan without these kinds of compensation arrangements is difficult. Having your doctor responsible for a medical budget is not wrong, but you need to understand the compensation system and develop a trusting relationship with your doctor whatever the system.

The conflict between providing the best care and the incentives used to control costs in managed care can be a challenge for your doctor. Many physicians receive the majority of their patients from one or more managed care organizations. Some doctors are concerned that if they confront a managed care organization's procedures and policies on behalf of patients, they may be risking their relationship with the organization. Nonetheless, the ethic of the Hippocratic Oath still prevails and your doctor is professionally and morally bound to do what is best for you.

How much the doctor is legally bound to do what is best for the patient may be changing, however. One of the ways in which managed care organizations significantly change the relationship between doctor and patient is to insert the insurer into it.

Insurer Makes Three

Under indemnity insurance you select a doctor, presumably for your lifetime. If you change plans it usually makes little difference, because doctors accept almost all indemnity insurance. Whatever the insurance doesn't pay, you, the patient, pay from your pocket. At the same time, indemnity insurers reimburse almost any doctor who is licensed to practice. In the indemnity system, selecting the provider is the patient's role; paying the bill is the insurer's role.

In managed care the insurer plays a role in selecting your doctor by limiting your choice to those it has selected to be part of its network. If you change managed care plans, you may have to change doctors if your doctor is not part of your new plan's network. At the same time, if your doctor leaves your plan you cannot follow (except when you change plans) because your contractual relationship is with the HMO, which must provide another doctor to care for you.

This is a significant change and one patients and doctors frequently dislike. Unfortunately, it is part of the new world of managed care.

Most doctors dislike managed care. A recent survey conducted by the American Medical Association (AMA) found that 92 percent of the doctors polled felt that managed care had a negative impact on their clinical independence; 81 percent also felt it had a negative impact on the patient-physician relationship, and 71 percent a negative impact on quality of care. Managed care forces doctors to discount their traditional fees or accept other compensation arrangements that are different and usually more restrictive than fee-for-service. In 1995, for the first time since the data has been gathered, the real income of doctors decreased! Many believe managed care is the primary reason.

Managed care health plans also monitor doctors, something most doctors are not used to, by measuring adherence to procedures and/or guidelines and by measuring patient satisfaction. It is not difficult to

NEARLY TWO PHYSICIANS IN FIVE (38 PERCENT) REPORT THAT THEIR ABILITY TO MAKE DECISIONS THEY THINK ARE RIGHT FOR THEIR PATIENTS HAS DECLINED IN THE PAST THREE YEARS, ACCORDING TO A REPORT BY THE COMMONWEALTH FUND.

understand why doctors do not like a system that restricts the way they practice, reduces their fees, more closely monitors their activities, and, in the opinion of some, reduces their patients' access to and quality of care.

On the other hand, much of this monitoring benefits patients. For example, Physician's Health Services (PHS), a leading Connecticut-based HMO, has a very extensive physician practice profile which deals with issues such as member satisfaction, reviews of office settings, continuing medical education, delivery of preventive services, and availability to patients. PHS uses these assessments to work with its physicians to improve the delivery of care. Many other HMOs follow similar practices.

When managed care first moves into an area doctors usually resist it. Most would prefer to continue their practices in a fee-for-service setting without the constraints of managed care. However, when managed care begins to control large segments of the health care market (and in many communities managed care enrolls 50-60 percent of the insured population) doctors have little choice but to sign on with managed care.

Some doctors not only resist, but resist strongly. Some have organized unions to bargain with managed care and some have formed other kinds of associations to oppose managed care. A group of physicians in New York State has adopted the name Code Blue (which in medicine indicates a patient has gone into cardiac arrest) to assist consumers who need help dealing with problems with their managed health care plans. Physicians Who Care is a national organization with the same purpose; their phone number is (800) 545-9305.

Despite the resistance and even outright hostility to managed care exhibited by many doctors, the medical profession is making adjustments to what is for it also a new reality. A 1997 survey by the American College of Physicians found that 57 percent of doctors surveyed indicated that they were either satisfied (47 percent) or very satisfied (10 percent) with the managed care organization with whom they were affiliated.

Today, approximately 85 percent of doctors have arrangements with at least one managed care organization. This clearly refutes the old notion that the best doctors don't participate in managed care. The new reality is that almost all doctors participate in managed care!

TO COMBAT RISING DRUG COSTS — UP ABOUT 13 PER-CENT IN 1996 — SOME HMOS ARE PUTTING PHYSICIANS ON BUDGETS FOR DRUGS, WHERE THE DOCTORS ARE AT RISK, ACCORDING TO A *NEW YORK TIMES* ARTICLE.

•Issues and Controversy•

Outpatient Mastectomies

Similar in nature to "Drive-through Births" is the issue of outpatient mastectomies. While it is true that most lumpectomies are performed on an outpatient basis, the notion of sending home women who had a portion of their breast removed, with tubes still inserted, was not a popular one. About 7.6 percent of mastectomies were done on an outpatient basis in 1995. The brouhaha developed when some Connecticut physicians complained that two area HMOs were *requiring* outpatient mastectomies. While the plans denied it, it was clear there was pressure to limit hospital stays for mastectomy patients and the ensuing outcry was loud and instant. Legislation was introduced into Congress, and in many states, requiring at least a 48 hour hospital stay after a mastectomy.

The American Association of Health Plans rapidly responded with this policy statement: "Health plans do not and should not require outpatient care for removal of a breast. Decisions about a hospital stay following mastectomy should be made by a woman's physician in consultation with the patient herself."

Again, managed care as an industry had to recover from the impression that profits were more important than patients and convince the public and political leaders that actual decisions would be made by doctors based on the needs of their patients.

There is little question that both "Drive-through Births" and outpatient mastectomies did irreparable harm to the managed care industry and prompted state and federal legislators to become even more assertive in their efforts to control many aspects of managed care through legislation.

Notes & Phone Numbers

_____

_____

_____

_____

_____

_____

_____

_____

_____

_____

_____

_____

_____

_____

_____

_____

Part Four

SPECIAL
CONSIDERATIONS

Highlights 11

Each year more Americans who receive Medicare join HMOs. Like other Americans, they are concerned about quality and choice, as well as their own special health care needs.

QUESTIONS ANSWERED IN THIS CHAPTER INCLUDE:

Do all HMOs take Medicare recipients?

Which is better, an HMO or Medigap insurance?

Can you get quality care in a Medicare HMO?

What issues should mature Americans consider when choosing a managed care health plan?

If I live in Chicago for six months, and Florida for six months, will my HMO provide coverage in both places?

Medigap or Managed Care

CHOICES FOR MATURE AMERICANS

Perhaps more than any other socioeconomic group, older adults need to be particularly cautious and informed when selecting an HMO. Because they are more likely to need medical attention, those 65 years and older stand to lose more if their health plan is too limited. Average life expectancy in 1900 was only 47 years. Today it is 76 years. The fastest growing age group of our population is those over 85. The fact that so many of us will be living longer than our forebears introduces a whole new set of health care concerns hardly known in previous centuries. Arthritis, cancer, heart disease, and dementia were as rare in the last century as a 60th birthday. Even the loss of physical strength or the inability to keep up with everyday chores such as cleaning, shopping, or cooking can hinder a healthy or independent existence.

While aging doesn't have to mean illness or a restricted lifestyle, there are, obviously, problems associated with getting older that, if not preventable, can at least be prepared for. Choosing the right health care coverage before you are confronted with any of these problems can help to make those later years healthier and happier.

On the average, older Americans spend four times more for health services than their younger counterparts. Most of these costs are covered by Medicare, the federally sponsored health insurance program for the disabled and those over the age of 65. In fact, more than 97 percent of older Americans are insured primarily by Medicare. While most Medicare beneficiaries rely on the financial security and access to health care that Medicare provides, the potential for large out-of-pocket expenses for health care exists. According to the Office of the Actuary at the Health Care Financing Administration, these costs can average 14 percent of an older person's disposable income as compared with only 4 percent for the non-elderly. In general, Medicare requires beneficiaries to pay 20 percent of covered medical services as well as hospital deductibles, copayments, premiums, and the cost of outpatient prescription drugs. Medicare does not cover most institutional long-term care.

What Are the Options?

For those who are relatively healthy, basic Medicare coverage alone may be sufficient. But for many people, especially those with serious or chronic illnesses, the costs incurred by the individual or family can wipe out a life's savings rather quickly. Even without serious or chronic illness, most Medicare recipients recognize the utility of subscribing to Medicare Part B, presently at $43.80 a month, to cover doctor visits, diagnostic tests, lab services, and home health care.

To address additional gaps in coverage, such as out-of-pocket costs, prescription drugs, or eyeglasses, private insurance to supplement Medicare is available in the form of Medigap policies. There are 10 such standardized policies, lettered A (the basic plan) through J, although not all of the policies are available in all states, and prices may vary from insurer to insurer. However, each individual plan is identical from insurer to insurer, regardless of cost.

Obviously, the more coverage you want, the more it is going to cost. Depending on where you live, the basic plan, A, may cost as little as $300 to $400 a year and plan J, the most comprehensive, can cost more than $2,800 a year.

Keep in mind that insurers are prohibited from checking on the health of new applicants age 65 and older for six months after they sign up for Medicare Part B (medical services). So if you have any type of chronic illness, it's important to buy a Medicare supplement policy *before* the six months are up. Otherwise, you may find it difficult and expensive to obtain any insurance coverage. If you're already covered under a Medigap policy and are satisfied with your coverage, you don't have to switch to a new plan, particularly if your current policy pays for such amenities as private duty nurses. The new plans no longer provide coverage for these services.

MANAGED MEDICARE PLANS ENROLL MORE PEOPLE WITH INCOMES BELOW $30,000 THAN DO FEE-FOR-SERVICE PROGRAMS.

Choosing an HMO

Medigap policies are not the only way to go when looking to supplement your Medicare coverage. In fact, as with the population in general, the future for Medicare beneficiaries seems to point toward managed care. Historically, enrollment of Medicare beneficiaries in managed care has lagged behind the private sector. In recent years, however, enrollment among all HMOs increased substantially and currently more than 12 percent of Medicare beneficiaries are enrolled in managed care options — and they are joining HMOs at the rate of 80,000 a month! The number of managed care plans offering Medicare eligible services now numbers more than 330.

Many private employers are encouraging their retirees to join Medicare HMOs because they save money as compared to indemnity plans. Medicare recipients can also save money, and often receive additional benefits such as prescription drugs and eyeglasses, if they make the switch from many of the Medigap plans to a Medicare HMO.

All this is to say that many HMOs can serve to fill in the gaps of Medicare coverage. Whether or not these HMOs are better than Medigap policies depends upon your needs and the HMO. The advantages of HMOs are that they can be less expensive than conventional insurance plans, they may provide all your medical care in one place, and they may offer more services than those traditionally covered under Medicare. On the other hand, some recipients don't like having their choice of doctors and hospitals restricted. Also, HMOs are not yet policed as rigidly as traditional insurance providers. As a result, some HMOs can make receiving certain costly benefits, such as skilled nursing or home care, difficult for the elderly. According to *Consumer Reports*, some HMOs have been known to drag out the process of paying for these benefits so long that Medicare beneficiaries have died before ever receiving care they were legally entitled to! The trick is to choose a high quality HMO. One thing is clearly in the favor of HMOs: They reduce paperwork by eliminating claim forms as well as deductibles and co-insurance in most cases. They also tend to offer broader coverages than indemnity plans.

HMOs that contract with Medicare to provide services to beneficiaries use one of three methods, which affect how members obtain medical services and what they pay for them. In the first method, known as risk contracts, Medicare pays the HMO a monthly sum to provide all the coverage for beneficiaries who join. The HMO is obligated to provide all Part A (hospital) and Part B (medical) services. In turn, the HMO usually charges members a monthly premium to cover the cost of Medicare deductibles and copayments. HMOs that offer risk contracts must take all applicants, regardless of their health, except those with end-stage kidney disease and those already in a Medicare hospice program. Members of risk contract HMOs are locked into using the HMO's services and are therefore not permitted to seek care outside of the network.

PRICE WATERHOUSE ECONOMISTS ESTIMATED THAT THE MEDICARE PROGRAM COULD SAVE $38.4 BILLION IF 40 PERCENT OF SENIORS SIGNED UP WITH HMOS. PRESENTLY ONLY 12 PERCENT OF SENIOR CITIZENS ARE ENROLLED IN HMOS.

In the second type of service provided by HMOs, known as cost contracts, Medicare pays the HMO a fee to provide hospital and medical services. As with risk contracts, the HMO charges monthly premiums that cover Medicare deductibles and copayments and must accept all older applicants. At the end of the year, if the plan has spent more than Medicare has paid, Medicare reimburses the HMO. Members belonging to an HMO using a cost contract method are not locked into the HMO; that is, they are free to seek medical services outside of the network. Medicare will reimburse them the cost of the care, but the beneficiary will then have to pay the usual copayments, deductibles, and extra doctors' charges.

Health care prepayment plans, the third contractual method, require that Medicare pays the HMO to provide medical services only, and not hospital services. The HMO does not have to cover all medical services but must provide for doctors' visits, X-rays, lab tests, and other diagnostic tests. Beneficiaries can go outside the plan for care, but again are responsible for any copayments, deductibles, and extra charges.

What to Look for

When you make any major decision, whether it be selecting a community for retirement or purchasing a home, you should first assess your needs and then research your options before making a selection. Choosing an HMO is no exception. You should make your selection only after carefully considering your current and future health care needs, your financial status, your preferences for physicians, hospitals and their locations, and matching these needs with an HMO's services.

At the age of 65, you may be robustly healthy, or you may have already had your share of health problems. While there are no crystal balls to predict what your health care future will bring, your past health care needs certainly should be considered when you're looking into an HMO. For example, if you've had a history of heart disease, you'll want to look for an HMO that provides comprehensive coverage in that area as well as a number of specialists and hospitals that are well regarded in that area of treatment. If you've developed a rapport with a physician and/or specialist who has treated you for a special health care problem in the past, you may want to find an HMO that includes him or her on its roster. Make sure that the HMO's physicians are conveniently located so you will be more likely to make and keep appointments.

> A PRIMARY CARE DOCTOR CAN TYPICALLY HANDLE 2,000 PATIENTS UNDER AGE 65 BUT ONLY 800 OVER 65.

Another issue of concern to many Medicare recipients is access to specialists. Check on the HMO's process for referrals to specialists. If you are seeing one regularly, for example a cardiologist, do you have to contact your primary care physician each time before you make an appointment?

Closely related to this is going outside the HMO network of providers. Is it possible for you to see a doctor who is not part of the network? If so, what is the process and the cost? If it is a POS (Point of Service) plan, you must still be certain to check out the procedure and cost of going out of network.

Once you've ascertained that an HMO can provide you with the core services that are important to you now, look into the variety and depth of other services provided. Perhaps one of the most important considerations seniors should take into account is coverage for long-term care. Because we are living longer, chances are that many of us will find ourselves needing some kind of long-term health care. Some 43 percent of Americans currently 65 or older are expected eventually to enter nursing homes, and more still will utilize the services of such other long-term care options as home care, adult day care, hospices, and assisted care. Ascertain what the extent of coverage is in each area for the HMO you are considering. Obviously, it is wise to find the most comprehensive coverage you can afford.

Although Medicare HMOs tend to offer broader coverages than many Medigap plans, they do not have standard benefit plans. Therefore, you need to review the specific coverages for such things as nursing home care, prescription drugs and limits on hospital days. In fact, review all coverages as outlined on pages 48-53!

Home care is another coverage to investigate carefully. The limits on home care vary by plan, sometimes significantly. Also, most coverages have caps or limits and they can vary. For example, a pharmacy benefit may have a $1,000 or $1,500 cap. Many of the POS plans have caps on how much they will pay for out-of-network care. The limits can range from $5,000 to $250,000.

Coverage when away from home is often another concern to Medicare recipients. In the past, and currently in some plans, Medicare HMO members were covered only for emergencies when traveling outside of their area, and even that benefit was limited to 90 days. For coverage during travel over 90 days, many HMO members canceled their membership and joined another plan temporarily.

New regulations governing Medicare now permit plans to offer coverage during travel for periods up to 12 months. However, HMOs differ in the coverages they offer, so check on it specifically.

Quality in HMO Medicare Plans

There has been some debate about quality, member selection, and government reimbursement in Medicare and managed care plans.

A 1996 study published in the *Journal of the American Medical Association* by John Ware of Boston's New England Medical Center concluded that the elderly and poor fared less well under managed care than indemnity insurance. Supporters of managed care have responded with a number of criticisms of the study, including noting that the measure of outcomes had

A SURVEY OF MEDICARE BENEFICIARIES IN ARIZONA, CALIFORNIA, FLORIDA AND TEXAS SHOWED OVER THREE-QUARTERS CHOSE HMOS BECAUSE THEY OFFERED MORE BENEFITS OR HAD LOWER COSTS.

only one dimension and that the data was old, collected between 1986 and 1990.

On the other hand, a survey of over 3,000 Medicare managed care enrollees showed they were satisfied with their plans. Conducted in 1996 for the Physician Payment Review Commission, the study found that only eight percent reported trouble seeing a physician and only six percent of those surveyed reported they had not been referred to a specialist if they wanted a specialist's care, or felt they had been discharged from the hospital too soon. Only four percent of the respondents labeled their care "fair" or "poor." Medicare HMOs scored well on preventive services such as flu shots and mammograms.

There is a shortage of studies regarding the outcomes and satisfaction of Medicare HMO members. The general rule should be to follow all of the methods we have listed to determine quality in plans you are considering.

The quality of HMO Medicare plans is often reflected in their disenrollment rates. One study showed these can range from four percent to 42 percent. The data on disenrollment rates is not easy to obtain but can be secured from the Health Care Financing Agency (HCFA) of the federal government through the Freedom of Information Act. It is not a simple process, but may be well worth it.

The federal government is currently reviewing many of the regulations governing Medicare HMOs. Included among forthcoming changes are a time limit of 72 hours for resolving most appeals in cases affecting the lives, health, or maximum function of recipients. Currently, HMOs have as long as 60 days to resolve these complaints. The changes will also give Medicare recipients the right to appeal reductions in benefits, as well as the right to appeal any reduction in care.

Another issue the federal government is considering is a reduction in the amount paid to Medicare HMOs. At present the government reimburses 95 percent of the estimated cost for caring for similar patients in the same geographic area under fee-for-service Medicare programs. Some have claimed the Medicare HMOs enroll generally healthier patients and, as a result, are being over-compensated for care. The American Association of Health Plans, the group that represents HMOs and other managed care organizations, claims that there is no difference in the health status of the people enrolled in a Medicare HMO and non-HMO. Many seniors are concerned that a reduction in reimbursement rates could lead to a reduction in benefits.

A concluding note: If you are shifting from Medigap insurance for a few months, make sure you get the coverage you need. If you drop your Medigap plan it could be more difficult to re-enroll, especially if you have a chronic disease.

NINETY-SIX PERCENT OF MEDICARE HMO MEMBERS RATED THEIR CARE AS GOOD OR EXCELLENT, IN A STUDY COMMISSIONED BY THE PHYSICIAN PAYMENT REVIEW COMMISSION.

•Issues and Controversy•

Denial of Care

Perhaps the most frightening issue to consumers, and the one that has attracted major press and political attention, is that of being denied care. There have been some highly visible cases and lawsuits that have attracted tremendous media publicity. These cases are naturals for media exploitation. They involve a sick or dying person and a large company with millions of dollars in revenue saying it will not pay for a treatment that may save the person's life. Unfortunately, these cases always have and always will be with us. Indemnity insurers also deny care to people they insure and they do it for the same reason managed care organizations do: In most cases, the care desired is not covered by the insured person's policy. Also, insurance companies of all kinds typically deny reimbursement for care they deem as experimental. They also deny care if they believe it would be ineffective or wasteful. They are often slow — perhaps too slow — to reimburse for new treatments until they are widely accepted. But this is not just a managed care issue; it's an indemnity insurance issue as well.

This issue was vividly dramatized by the case of a California woman who sued her HMO because it denied a bone marrow transplant to combat breast cancer. Some experts claimed the therapy was still unproven. Other experts claimed it would help — perhaps save the woman's life. Some insurers reimburse for the procedure, others do not. Whether effective or not, the question is moot: The woman died after her HMO refused to pay for a bone marrow transplant and her estate was awarded $89.1 million when it sued the HMO!

Exclusions are a far simpler issue. Some procedures and treatments, such as cosmetic surgery, chiropractic care, sex-change operations, and dental care, are frequently not covered. Not to be denied, however, some patients and some providers (like chiropractors) are asking the courts or state legislatures to mandate by law coverage for certain kinds of care. Nonetheless, if the contract excludes it, the HMO has no obligation to pay.

Although these examples tend to grab the headlines, there is another, less dramatic kind of denial of care that troubles many people. This kind of denial concerns the patient who wants to have another test or another procedure; the patient who wants to be certain that every avenue has been explored, every option taken to either diagnose or solve a problem. Perhaps the most common and most annoying kind of denial concerns referrals to specialists. This is a major issue for many HMO members and doctors. Frequently a primary care physician's referral to another specialist has to be reviewed and approved. Since restricting ready access to specialists is one of the major ways HMOs control costs, the criticism has been intense and often public. Many HMOs have eased referrals to specialists by not reviewing referrals made by a primary care physicians. Is the denial based on honest medical opinion that an additional test or procedure is unnecessary and even wasteful, or is it based on a desire primarily to control costs, either on the part of the HMO or the doctor, or both?

A related question is "who is making the decision?" Is it your doctor, or another doctor hundreds of miles away who has never examined you but is a "medical director"? This issue concerns not only doctors but patients. However, in managed care plans, and even in indemnity programs these days, such oversight and review procedures are common.

This issue demonstrates why members of an HMO must be assertive, knowledgeable and have confidence their doctor will do what is best for them, despite the financial incentives to the contrary. You should ask your insurer and your doctor to explain their policy on treatment you may feel you could need at some future time, including any financial incentives they have to withhold care. If denied access to a test or procedure, you should ask your doctor why it was denied and whether he or she supports the decision. If you are not satisfied with the responses, you should appeal to the HMO. If still denied, it may be better to pay for the test or procedure yourself and then appeal to the state insurance department or the courts to determine who should pay ultimately.

Notes & Phone Numbers

Highlights 12

Medical emergencies have been an issue of some controversy in managed care. There is often confusion about when it is correct to go to the emergency room.

QUESTIONS ANSWERED IN THIS CHAPTER INCLUDE:

What is the proper way to use the emergency department?

Do I have to pay if I use emergency services?

What happens if I have a medical emergency when I am traveling out of the area covered by my health plan?

Emergencies

CRITICAL CHOICES AT CRITICAL TIMES

A frequent issue in HMOs relates to payments for visits to emergency rooms. One of the problems under indemnity insurance is that some people use the hospital emergency department as their primary care doctor. If they have an upset stomach, a severe headache, a sore back — anything — they go to the emergency room for treatment. Because hospitals can bill whatever they choose for providing such care, it is an expensive form of care, and HMOs have done their best to minimize it. The way HMOs have attacked the problem is a simple one. They require you to call or use your primary care doctor first. If he okays your visit to the emergency department of a hospital, fine. If not, you visit the doctor, not the hospital.

Of course, in life-threatening or real emergencies (e.g. a heart attack or a broken limb), you can go to the emergency department directly, without prior authorization from your primary care doctor or a manager at the HMO.

The problem is that all too frequently patients believe their condition warrants emergency care, but the HMO does not agree. Of course, some patients simply forget to call the HMO for prior authorization and they understandably get the bill.

CASE STUDY

Dwight Moller traveled a great deal in his job. On a recent trip to Chicago, however, he became terribly ill. He had indigestion, nausea, and a tightness in his chest. He was afraid he was having a heart attack, since he was overweight, out of shape, and his family had a history of heart disease. Dwight's first thought was to go to the emergency room of the nearest hospital, but he remembered his health plan had an emergency assistance number. He called it and was directed to a different hospital, a little further away, that was under contract to provide emergency coverage for his plan.

It turned out his problem was severe gastrointestinal distress. He received excellent care, and he only paid a small copay. Had he visited the emergency room he initially wanted to use, he could have ended up paying the entire bill! ∎

However, the patient who is really sick and *feels* as if he or she is dying, even if he or she is not, is reluctant to pay a bill he or she feels the HMO should pay. This frequently causes a problem for hospitals, who end up getting stuck for the bill because neither the HMO nor the patient wants to pay.

Another way HMOs have attempted to reduce the use of emergency departments is to require a copayment of $25 to $35 for each visit to the emergency department. However, one study found that while this reduced emergency department visits by 15 percent, some patients who decided not to go had serious problems that would have been classified as emergencies!

The American College of Emergency Physicians has recommended federal standards for emergency room situations. Together with Kaiser Permanente, the nation's largest HMO, they have called for legislation that would require insurers to make payment decisions based on symptoms, rather than on the ultimate diagnosis. Specifically, the legislation would mandate payment if a "prudent layperson" could reasonably expect his or her condition to result in serious health impairment. The proposed legislation would also require emergency room physicians to contact the HMO within 30 minutes after a patient is stabilized to consult on the next step.

The "prudent layperson" standard, which some states have adopted, makes a strong case for patient participation in his or her own health care. This is not to say that patients should be required to diagnose their own conditions; however, it does imply that patients must give some serious consideration to the severity of symptoms before dashing off to an emergency room.

Out-of-Area Coverage

The issue of out-of-area coverage is related to that of emergencies. Some people have run into problems because their HMO pays for coverage only within the network. If you are out of the area and are sick, you either travel back to your home to be treated or you pay for treatment yourself.

True medical emergencies that occur out-of-area are covered, of course. But again, the issue becomes one of definition. When is something a true medical emergency? Some HMOs have arrangements with other HMOs, or with networks of hospitals around the country, to provide emergency care for their members. Many HMOs require a member to return to a network hospital and network doctors for follow-up care once the emergency has passed. It's wise to know this in advance. It is important for you to know what the rules are and follow them. Check this out before you enroll (if you have a choice) or, at least, before you travel. If you are traveling internationally there are insurance policies you can purchase that will provide care or return you home for care.

OF CALLERS TO NURSE CALL LINES, ONLY TWO PERCENT ARE STEERED TO EMERGENCY ROOMS, AND ABOUT 15 PER-CENT TO URGENT CARE, ACCORDING TO A *WALL STREET JOURNAL* ARTICLE.

Highlights 13

A brief look forward is especially appropriate because of the rapid changes in health care today.

QUESTIONS ANSWERED IN THIS CHAPTER INCLUDE:

How will managed care change in the future?

Will the controversial issues we have read about and heard continue to be problems?

What will be the impact of all the legislative activity?

Will managed care limit my choices or increase them in the future?

Looking Ahead

WHERE DO WE GO FROM HERE?

This book contains a great deal of information. Although we have tried to present it in a simple and interesting fashion, all the advice we offer on choosing a plan may entail more effort than you wish to expend. Hopefully not, because your ability to get the best health care will be directly related (unless you are simply lucky) to the effort you make to find the best health plan, best doctors and best hospitals.

Most people spend a great deal of time and effort planning vacations, buying a car, or even choosing a restaurant for an evening out. Why not spend a similar amount selecting the best health plan for yourself and your family?

This concluding chapter has two parts. First, a look forward: What can we, as consumers and patients, expect in the next few years? One thing is certain: consumers will need to play a more assertive role in finding the best care. Second, a brief summary, in outline form, that you can use as a guide in selecting a health plan. Use it in conjunction with the various parts of this book and it should be extremely helpful. Also, don't forget to review the appendices. They contain a great deal of useful information.

What's Ahead

The environment for managed care is, in large measure, driven by competition with indemnity insurance and has been based primarily on cost. Both the government's and private employers' first concern has been cost, not quality. Managed care clearly has won the battle with indemnity insurance and now dominates most markets. However, that victory has had a price: major concerns about quality from consumers, the government, employers, and the media. As a result, the field of competition is changing from competing with indemnity insurance to competition among HMOs, and from competition based on price to competition based on quality. Although price will always be an important principle in this new era of competition, quality, and the perception of quality, will become paramount. As managed indemnity tries to tighten controls on costs and managed care attempts to give consumers more choices, they will become less distinguishable. The health care environment is still in a state of rapid change. As a result, managed health plans will make serious efforts, primarily through quality of care and service, and by marketing quality, to distinguish themselves and create brand recognition.

Managed care organizations will continue to merge and grow larger. One reason for this is that despite the perception of these organizations growing rich, the majority *lost* money in 1996.

As managed care grows larger, so will systems of hospitals and networks of physicians, driven by the necessity to provide large networks to serve regional and national health plans. American health care is becoming ever more corporatized.

Outpatient care will continue to grow, and weaker hospitals will close. Those that remain will differentiate their programs. In large systems or networks, individual hospitals will not try to be all things to all people; they will specialize and share in attempts to reduce their costs to compete and to survive.

The challenges are almost as great for doctors as they are for hospitals. The growth in managed care has reduced the need for specialists and increased the need for primary care physicians. Physicians find their incomes lagging and their control over their profession diminishing.

Consumers face new challenges as well. It is becoming clear that consumers need to be better informed about their choices in health plans. They know how critical those choices can be. As a result they, and those who pay for most of our health care (the government and employers), are demanding more information, especially ratings of plans by other consumers and true outcomes studies.

As a result of some of the managed care horror stories we have heard, read, and seen, government at both state and federal levels is taking an active posture towards the regulation of managed care. Over 400 bills aimed at controlling various aspects of managed care were submitted in over 40 states in 1996. Over 1,000

A KAISER FAMILY FOUNDATION SURVEY SHOWED THAT OVER ONE-HALF OF THE VOTERS SURVEYED FELT THE GOVERNMENT NEEDED TO PROTECT CONSUMERS FROM BEING TREATED UNFAIRLY AND NOT GETTING THE CARE THEY SHOULD FROM MANAGED CARE PLANS.

bills have been submitted in 1997.

These bills deal with virtually every issue of contention in managed care: access to specialists; emergency care; denials of care; births; mastectomies; hospital stays; physician payments; appeals; gag rules; and willing provider issues. Some of these bills are designed to protect patients, some to protect providers. Some are proposed because they make good press rather than deal rationally with complex medical issues. Others are serious attempts to prevent abuses. Nonetheless, they do pose a threat to managed care and promise not only continued scrutiny, but also the risk of micromanagement by state legislatures or Congress.

The result of this legislative interest and activity undoubtedly will be stronger laws protecting consumers. Already a number of regulations have modified how managed care organizations deal with their members. Gag rules have been removed, appeals procedures strengthened, limits have been placed on patient discharges and other measures are being considered by the federal and state governments to protect consumers. Perhaps the most serious threat to managed care are laws designed to eliminate ERISA protections and permit members to sue MCOs.

The managed care industry has responded with its own patient protection initiative, labeled "Putting Patients First," which the American Association of Health Plans has adopted. In an attempt to respond to payer and consumer concerns, as well as to head off, as much as possible, the legislative efforts to control managed care, the AAHP spelled out several policies for its members on issues that often have been troubling to the public. Putting Patients First requires plans to provide patients with information about how participating physicians will be paid; on utilization review procedures; on the basis for specific utilization review decisions; whether a specific prescription drug is included in the formulary; and how the plan decides when a treatment or procedure is considered experimental.

Despite the efforts of both government and the managed care industry, the burden of responsibility still rests heavily on individuals. The best intended legislation cannot ensure quality care. The most well-meaning manager cannot approve payment of a bill for services not covered in a plan. The most supportive state agency cannot help you get care if you need it urgently.

Consumers have to choose the best plans, know their policies and rules well, and be assertive in demanding the best. Only then can managed care health plans deliver their promise of providing quality care, while still controlling costs.

The outline which follows can be used by itself or, even better, in conjunction with the material in the text of this book, as a quick checklist to assist you in selecting the best health plan. Remember that choice varies by individual and by family. Choose the plan that meets *your* particular needs.

IN CHOOSING A HEALTH PLAN, AMERICANS SAY QUALITY OF CARE IS THEIR PRIMARY CONCERN (42 PERCENT) FOLLOWED BY COST (18 PERCENT), A WIDE CHOICE OF DOCTORS (17 PERCENT), AND A RANGE OF BENEFITS (14 PERCENT), ACCORDING TO A SURVEY BY THE KAISER FAMILY FOUNDATION AND THE AGENCY FOR HEALTH CARE POLICY AND RESEARCH.

Questions & Answers
HMO Checklist

The following questions will provide you with a quick "checklist" to use as a guide or reminder in the process of selecting an HMO or other managed care plan. Make certain you have found out the answers to, or a least considered, the following questions! Beside each question the chapter where information and explanations can be found is noted.

Do you know what model the HMO is? Chapter 4

What is the premium cost each month?
To you? To your employer? Chapter 6

Are there copays? When? How much? Chapter 6

Is there a deductible? What is the amount?
Individual? Family? Chapter 6

How do you enroll? When? When can you change? Chapter 3

If you're being insured through your employer, who
in the company is your contact to answer questions? Chapter 3

Have you reviewed the quality of the health plan? Chapter 7

    Accreditation? Chapter 7

    Provider network? Chapter 7

    Satisfaction surveys? Chapter 7

    Outcomes studies? Chapter 7

CHAPTER THIRTEEN

Are there other providers in the network such as pharmacies, rehab centers, etc? Are they accessible and of good quality?	Chapter 7
Is the network of doctors large and does it contain a sufficient selection of primary care and other specialists so you have reasonable choices?	Chapters 7 & 10
How do you choose doctors, primary care and other specialists? How, and when, can you change doctors?	Chapters 5 & 10
How are you referred to a specialist? Do you have choices?	Chapters 7 & 10
If you want a second opinion how is that permitted? Arranged?	Chapters 7 & 10
In what specialty is your primary care doctor trained?	Chapters 5 & 9
Is he/she board certified?	Chapters 7 & 9
What is the waiting time for appointments?	Chapter 7
How is your doctor compensated? Are there set-asides? Capitation?	Chapter 8
What is the appeals process in the health plan?	Chapter 9

Appendices

Notes & Phone Numbers

Appendix A

RATING HMO COVERAGES
BASED ON FAMILY NEEDS

The purpose of this format is for you to rate the coverages offered by the health plan you are considering. This structure will assist you in making comparisons. The numerical totals should not be viewed as absolutes; rather, they should serve as a guide for you in selecting a plan.

Rating - Rate each coverage: 3 = excellent, 2 = good, 1 = poor. Use the high end and low end examples, as well as coverages in other plans, as a guide to make these judgements.

Family Needs - Some coverages are more important to families than others. Rate the importance of this coverage to your family: 3 = very important, 2 = somewhat important, 1 = not important.

Multiply the rating by the family needs value to determine the total score for that coverage. Add up all the total scores to get the grand total for that HMO. **Example:**

Benefit	Rating of Coverage	Importance to Family	Total Score
PHYSICAL EXAMS	3 **X**	2	= 6

Plan Form

Plan Name_____

Benefit	Rating of Coverage	Importance to Family	Total Score
ALLERGY TESTS & TREATMENTS	X	=	
ALTERNATIVE CARE (ACUPUNCTURE CHIROPRACTIC CARE, MASSAGE THERAPY, NATUROPATHY, NUTRITIONISTS & DIETITIANS, YOGA)	X	=	
AMBULANCE SERVICES	X	=	
AREA OF SERVICE	X	=	
CONSULTATIONS	X	=	
DENTAL CARE	X	=	
DEPENDENT DEFINITION	X	=	
DIAGNOSTIC TESTS (CAT SCAN, MRI, X-RAY, CLINICAL LABORATORY)	X	=	
DURABLE MEDICAL EQUIPMENT	X	=	
EAR & EYE EXAMS	X	=	
EMERGENCY/URGENT CARE	X	=	
EXPERIMENTAL TREATMENT	X	=	
EXTENDED CARE	X	=	
FAMILY PLANNING (CONTRACEPTIVES, ELECTIVE ABORTION, NATURAL FAMILY PLANNING, TUBAL LIGATION, VASECTOMY)	X	=	
HEARING AIDS	X	=	
HOME HEALTH CARE	X	=	
HOSPICE CARE	X	=	
INFERTILITY	X	=	
MAMMOGRAMS	X	=	
MAXIMUM LIFETIME COVERAGE	X	=	
MENTAL HEALTH – INPATIENT	X	=	
MENTAL HEALTH – OUTPATIENT	X	=	
OCCUPATIONAL THERAPY – INPATIENT	X	=	

OCCUPATIONAL THERAPY – OUTPATIENT	X	=
ORGAN TRANSPLANTS	X	=
OUT-OF-NETWORK CARE	X	=
OUTSIDE SECOND OPINION	X	=
PHYSICAL EXAMS	X	=
PHYSICAL THERAPY – INPATIENT	X	=
PHYSICAL THERAPY – OUTPATIENT	X	=
PODIATRY	X	=
PRE-EXISTING CONDITIONS	X	=
PRENATAL CARE (INCLUDING AMNIOCENTESIS, CHORIONIC VILLI SAMPLING, ULTRASOUND)	X	=
PRESCRIPTION DRUGS	X	=
PROSTHETICS	X	=
SKILLED NURSING CARE	X	=
SPEECH THERAPY – INPATIENT	X	=
SPEECH THERAPY – OUTPATIENT	X	=
SUBSTANCE ABUSE – INPATIENT	X	=
SUBSTANCE ABUSE – OUTPATIENT	X	=
SURGERY	X	=
VISION	X	=
WELL-BABY CARE	X	=
WELLNESS PROGRAMS	X	=

Grand Total _____

Notes & Phone Numbers

Appendix B

STATE AGENCIES REGULATING HMOs

The following are the phone numbers of the state agencies that regulate HMOs.

ALABAMA	(334) 269-3550
ALASKA	none
ARIZONA	(602) 912-8400
ARKANSAS	(501) 371-2600
CALIFORNIA	(916) 654-8076
COLORADO	(303) 894-7499
CONNECTICUT	(860) 297-3800
DELAWARE	(302) 577-3119
state residents only	(800) 282-8611
DISTRICT OF COLUMBIA	(202) 727-8000
FLORIDA	(904) 922-3131
GEORGIA	(404) 656-2056
HAWAII	(808) 586-4077

IDAHO	(208) 334-2250
ILLINOIS	(217) 492-4104
INDIANA	(317) 232-2385
IOWA	(515) 281-5705
KANSAS	(913) 296-3071
KENTUCKY	(502) 564-3630
LOUISIANA	(504) 342-5900
MAINE	(207) 624-8475
MARYLAND	(410) 468-2000
MASSACHUSETTS	(617) 521-7794
MICHIGAN	(517) 373-0240
MINNESOTA	(612) 296-4026
MISSISSIPPI	(601) 359-3569
MISSOURI *or*	(800) 726-7390 (573) 751-4126
MONTANA	(800) 332-6148
NEBRASKA	(402) 471-2201
NEVADA	(702) 687-4270
NEW HAMPSHIRE	(603) 271-2261
NEW JERSEY	(609) 292-5360
NEW MEXICO	(505) 827-4500

NEW YORK
state residents only   (800) 342-3736

NORTH CAROLINA   (919) 733-7343

NORTH DAKOTA   (701) 328-2440

OHIO   (614) 644-2673
state residents only   (800) 686-1526

OKLAHOMA   (405) 271-6868
state residents only   (800) 811-4552 *(ans. machine)*

OREGON   (503) 947-7984

PENNSYLVANIA   (717) 787-2317

RHODE ISLAND   (401) 277-2223

SOUTH CAROLINA   (803) 737-6160

SOUTH DAKOTA   (605) 773-3563

TENNESSEE   (615) 741-2218
state residents only   (800) 342-4029

TEXAS   (512) 322-4266
state residents only   (800) 252-3439 *(for complaints only)*

UTAH   (801) 538-3800

VERMONT   (802) 828-3302

VIRGINIA   (804) 371-9741

WASHINGTON   (360)753-7300
state residents only   (800) 562-6900

WEST VIRGINIA   (304) 558-3386
state residents only   (800) 642-9004

WISCONSIN	(608) 266-3585
WYOMING	(307) 777-7401

Appendix C

CONSUMER SURVEYS AND RATINGS OF HMOs

Boston Magazine: "Is Your HMO a Dog" (http://www.bostonmagazine.com)

Boston Magazine has reports available on their website about Massachusetts HMOs. Compiled from surveys distributed by the New England HEDIS Coalition, the ratings measure consumer satisfaction in response to the following questions:

- Overall, how would you evaluate health care at your plan?

- Access to medical care when you need it?

- Thoroughness of exam and accuracy of diagnosis?

- Ease of seeing the doctor of your choice?

- Personal interest in you and your medical problems?

- The outcomes of your health care. How much were you helped?

- Would you recommend your health insurance plan to your family or friends if they needed help?

- Do you intend to switch to a different health plan when you next have an opportunity?

The plans covered were: Community Health Plans, Central Massachusetts Health Care, Fallon Community Health Plans, Harvard Community Health Plans, Health New England, Bay State, HMO Blue, HealthSource

New Hampshire, Kaiser Permanente, Matthew Thornton Health Plan, Neighborhood Health Plan, Pilgrim Health Plan, Tufts Associated Health Plans, and US Healthcare.

Consumer Reports Magazine: "How Good is Your Health Plan?" (August, 1996)
CU/Reprints, 101 Truman Ave., Yonkers, NY 10703-1057

Consumer Reports surveyed plan members directly to compile their data on 51 of the best and worst HMOs (and 14 PPOs) in the nation, rather than rely on the plan-supplied HEDIS and report card data, which CR claims is misleading. To determine an "overall satisfaction score," CR rated HMOs by:

* Problems with care (not getting needed care)

* Satisfaction with doctors (availability, choice, and how the doctor relates to patients)

* Preventive medicine (reminders to get checkups/treatment, disease screenings)

The report also notes if the HMO is for-profit or not-for-profit, and its NCQA accreditation status. A separate chart rates PPOs along the same lines as the HMOs; there is also a chart that utilizes the HEDIS data to create a "preventive care" and "utilization" index for many of the plans.

The report concludes that not-for-profit HMOs are better at satisfying consumers than for-profit HMOs, and that NCQA accredited plans did not necessarily do a better job of satisfying consumers than non-accredited plans.

Newsweek: "Special Report: Does Your HMO Stand Up?" (June 24, 1996)
251 W 57th St., New York, NY 10019 (212) 445-4000

To rate the U.S.'s largest HMOs, *Newsweek*, in cooperation with the Foundation for Accountability, surveyed the HMOs themselves. Of the 75 HMOs surveyed, 43 responded. An overall score of one to four stars was then created by rating the HMOs in the following areas:

* Meets Industry Standards (Is it accredited, or planning to be accredit-

ed? Does it publish HEDIS data? Is it affiliated with JCAHO accredited hospitals? What is the percentage of doctors in the plan that are board certified?)

- Measures Satisfaction (Does the HMO measure member satisfaction? Does it measure the satisfaction of its doctors?)

- Tracks Members' Health (Does the plan do outcomes studies?)

- Prevention and Screening (Does the plan promote vaccination, mammography, cancer screening, etc.)

- Maternity Care (How many women received prenatal care in the first trimester? What percentage of deliveries are by C-section? What percentage of women with C-sections delivered normally afterwards?)

- Satisfied Customers (As provided by CareData; the Federal Center for the Study of Services; and a survey of a Fortune 500 companies' employees.)

- Complaints (Number of complaints per 10,000 members, as compared to the state average.)

The best plans, according to *Newsweek*, are those that have a close relationship with doctors and work to keep their members healthy.

U.S. News and World Report "Rating the HMOs" (September 2, 1996)
HMO Reprints, 2400 N Street NW, Washington, DC 20037-1196

The emphasis of the *U.S. News* report is on prevention. Using data from the NCQA, *U.S. News* created a "prevention index" based on how well each HMO met the federal goals for five different preventive measures: cholesterol screening, breast and cervical cancer screening, rate of childhood immunization, and share of pregnant women receiving care in the first trimester. The report has full information on 132 HMOs, and partial data on another 42 HMOs. The report gives the following data by state:

- *U.S. News* rating (1 to 4 stars)

- Prevention Score

- Percentage of members receiving the five preventive measures listed above.

- Accreditation status of the HMO.

- Percentage of primary care physicians and specialists in the HMO who are board certified.

- Annual turnover of physicians in the HMO.

- Total members in the HMO.

However, this additional data was not factored into the total rating, which was exclusively based on the prevention score of the HMO.

CareData Reports, Inc. (http://www.caredata.com)

CareData rates HMOs and PPOs, and provides downloadable reports from their website ($12.95 apiece). The HMOs and PPOs rated vary by region. Each report measures the following areas:

- Overall satisfaction

- Satisfaction with quality of medical care, overall.

- Satisfaction with choice of primary care physician.

- Overall satisfaction with specialists.

- Satisfaction with the quality and reputation of hospitals in the plan.

- Satisfaction with customer service.

The measures are based on surveys created by CareData and distributed by employers to their employees.

Appendix D

OTHER RESOURCES AND READINGS

Buyer's Guide to Managed Care
New York Business Group on Health, Inc., May, 1997
386 Park Avenue South, Suite 598, New York, NY 10016-8804 (212) 252-7440
$50.00

Explains the differences among the many kinds of managed care plans (HMO, PPO, POS). The heart of the *Buyer's Guide* is a comprehensive breakdown of the managed care plans in the New York City area, including rates, deductibles, number of primary care physicians and specialists, and type of plan. Also includes a glossary of managed care terms. The guide was written primarily for employers.

Consumer Coalition for Quality Health Care
1275 K Street NW, Suite 602, Washington, D.C. 20005 (202) 789-3606

A national, non-profit membership organization of consumer groups, the Consumer Coalition for Quality Health Care is dedicated to protecting and improving the quality of health care for all Americans. The Consumer Coalition works to ensure the quality of health care and to protect the rights of people in managed care plans. The Coalition works to increase the amount of information on health care, for stronger laws and regulations to protect health care consumers, and assists grassroots organizations in working for reforms at the state level. The Coalition's Quality Watchline, (800) 720-8090, is a hotline where consumers and health care workers can relate their experiences with poor quality health care. The

Coalition's webpage, http://www.consumers.org, serves as an introduction to the Coalition's agenda.

Consumer's Guide to Health Plans
Consumer's Checkbook, 1996.
733 15th St. NW, Suite 820, Washington, DC 20005 (202) 347-7283 $12.00

Details the different types of managed care, and provides guidelines to choosing an HMO. The *Consumer's Guide* also gives a state-by-state rating of consumer satisfaction with managed care providers in that state, compiled from a survey of federal employees. Other information includes data on the hospitals with the lowest death rates, and which state agencies to contact concerning managed care.

Facts About Managed Care
Business and Health Magazine, 1997
5 Paragon Dr., Montvale, NJ 07645-1742 (201) 358-7500 $49.00

Contains useful statistics on many different areas of managed care. Includes information on the percentage of HMOs using formularies; methods used to control costs; average cost and reimbursement for eye exams; and copayment requirements for outpatient prescriptions. Also includes a glossary of pharmaceutical terms related to managed care and a directory of managed care-related organizations.

Health Care CheckUp: Consumers at Risk
Consumer's Union, 1996
1666 Connecticut Ave., Suite 310, Washington, DC 20009-1039 (202) 462-6262 $10.00

A critique of the current state of healthcare, *Consumers at Risk* criticizes the health care marketplace in general and managed care in particular. It charges that the decline in health care costs is not real, that consumers are getting less coverage for their money, and that managed care has actually increased the number of the uninsured, which will increase health costs for everyone. Includes recommendations for legislation to alleviate these problems.

Health Letter
Public Citizen Health Research Group
Circulation Department, 1600 20th Street NW, Washington, DC 20009

Founded by Ralph Nader and Dr. Sidney Wolfe, the Health Research

Group is a healthcare oriented consumer advocacy group. Their monthly newsletter, *Health Letter*, contains information on drugs, product recalls, current medical practices, and the state of the health care system (including managed care). The newsletter costs $18.00 for 12 issues.

Health Pages
135 Fifth Avenue, 7th floor, New York, NY, 10010

A monthly magazine that publishes separate editions in many major cities, *Health Pages* contains stories on all aspects of health care. Each month, a listing of physicians, HMOs, or hospitals is provided for the region covered by that edition. Available for $3.95 at newsstands or from the publisher.

HMO Consumers at Risk: States to the Rescue
Families USA, July, 1996
1334 G Street NW, Suite 300, Washington, DC 20005 (202) 628-3030 $15.00

Analyzing 14 key "protections," *States to the Rescue* helps to define exactly what you should expect from an HMO and which states provide the best enforcement to make sure you get the protection you need. Topics include: Access to, and coverage of, emergency treatment; state monitoring and oversight; grievances and complaint procedures for enrollees; and confidentiality of medical records. Includes an appendix detailing health care legislation enacted in the previous year, by state.

The Managed Care Consumer's Bill of Rights: A Health Policy Guide for Consumer Advocates
The Public Policy and Education Fund of New York
PPEF, 94 Central Ave., Albany, NY 12206 (518) 465-4600 $5.00

Rather than taking a stand on whether managed care is better or worse than traditional fee-for-service health care, the *Guide* suggests approaches to ensure customers get the most from managed care. Includes guidelines for pursuing claims against a managed care plan, and suggested legislation to ensure that a consumer's ten basic rights (access to care; choice of care; comprehensive benefits; affordability of care; quality of care; appeals; information; confidentiality and non-discrimination; representation; and enforcement) are protected.

People's Medical Society
462 Walnut Street, Allentown, PA 18102 (800) 624-8773

America's largest nonprofit consumer health advocacy organization, the People's Medical Society serves the public and its members by making available a wide variety of information on health care. Books, pamphlets, and the Society's monthly newsletter all help the consumer to become more informed and empowered in his or her health care decisions.

Source Book of Health Insurance Data
Health Insurance Association of America
555 13th St. NW, Washington, DC 20004 (202) 824-1600 $9.00

Organized in easy-to-read charts, the *Source Book of Health Insurance Data* provides a wealth of information on many aspects of health care, both under managed plans and fee-for-service, allowing quick comparisons to be made. Data include: average length of stay in a hospital, by procedure; health expenditure per enrollee in managed care plans; and personal health care expenses. Also includes a glossary of health care terms, and a chronology of managed care.

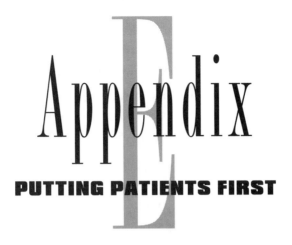

Appendix E

PUTTING PATIENTS FIRST

In December of 1996, the board of the American Association of Health Plans adopted a number of policy statements under the label "Patients First." In later modifications, additional policy statements were added and the title was changed to "Putting Patients First." The Board also announced, in March of 1997, that health plans joining or renewing memberships in the AAHP would be required to uphold the Association's patient-centered policies.

The following has been excerpted from Putting Patients First:

I. Patient's right to know

The Board of the AAHP stated that health plans should inform members about the plan's structure and provider network; benefits covered and excluded, including out-of-area and emergency coverage; and cost-sharing requirements, and should, upon request, inform a member about precertification and other utilization review procedures; the basis for a specific utilization review decision with which a member disagrees; whether a specific prescription drug is included in a formulary; a summary description of how participating physicians are paid, including financial incentive; (disclosure of specific details of financial arrangements should not be required); and the procedures and medically-based criteria a health plan uses to determine whether experimental treatments and technologies should become covered services, in the event of a dispute about coverage of such treatments and technologies.

II. Communications between patients and their physicians

At the same time, the Board adopted a statement affirming that nothing in any health plan policies or contracts between health plans and physicians should be interpreted as prohibiting physicians from discussing treatment options with patients.

III. Appeals and emergency care

In January of 1997, Putting Patients First addressed two issues that have been the source of considerable confusion: how health plans work with patients to resolve disputes over coverage or treatment decisions with which the patient disagrees, and how health plans cover and pay for emergency care while simultaneously discouraging unnecessary reliance on emergency facilities for non-emergency conditions:

- **Appeals:** Health plans should explain, in a timely notice to the patient, the basis for a coverage or treatment determination with which the patient disagrees, accompanied by an easily understood description of the patient's appeal rights and the time frames for an appeal. Appeals should be resolved as rapidly as warranted by the patient's situation. An expedited appeals process should be made available for situations in which the normal time frame could jeopardize a patient's life or health.

- **Emergency Care:** Health plans should cover emergency-room screening and stabilization as needed for conditions that reasonably appear to constitute an emergency, based on the patient's presenting symptoms. Emergency conditions are those that arise suddenly and require immediate treatment to avoid jeopardy to a patient's life or health. To promote continuity of care and optimal care by the treating physician, the emergency department should contact the patient's primary care physician as soon as possible.

In May of 1997 the AAHP board announced the following initiatives:

I. Physician-directed quality assessment and improvement programs

A unique advantage of health plans is that they have programs to assess and continually improve the quality of care available to members. Quality assessment and improvement programs should monitor targeted areas of patient care to detect whether patterns of underservice or overservice exist, and if so, to implement appropriate actions in order to promote access to the right care at the right time and in the right setting. The program should be physician-directed; participating physicians should be credentialed and periodically recredentialed; and all participating physicians should be informed of the program.

II. Physician-developed practice guidelines

Health plans rely on practice guidelines to promote appropriate care. Practice guidelines are intended to augment rather than supersede the physician-patient relationship by providing current scientific and medical information and decision-making support to practitioners, who are expected to offer patients their best professional judgement in light of this information based on their expertise and on the patient's individual circumstances. Practice guidelines should be based on current scientific and medical evidence; designed to involve participating physicians in their development and review; regularly updated; and available to participating physicians as appropriate to their specialty. An internal committee including participating physicians and other medical professionals with appropriate expertise should be available to consider requests from participating physicians that a guideline be modified based on relevant scientific medical evidence.

III. Physician-guided utilization management criteria

Because practice patterns and treatment recommendations can differ considerably from practitioner to practitioner and from area to area, utilization management—the process of making coverage determinations by evaluating the appropriateness of health care services—can play an important role in promoting consistently high-quality care at affordable cost.

Utilization management programs should be based on current scientific and medical evidence; should be directed by an experienced physician; and should involve participating physicians in reviewing utilization management criteria. Utilization management decisions should be based on clinical information about the patient, and the treating physician should have an opportunity to provide clinical information and the rationale for recommending a specific course of treatment prior to a utilization review determination. An exceptions process, directed by an experienced physician, should be available for cases in which a participating physician believes that a utilization management determination does not adequately account for the unique characteristics of a particular patient, based on relevant medical evidence offered by the participating physician for review.

IV. Physician-reviewed prescription drug formularies

Health plans develop formularies—lists of covered prescription drugs—to promote patients' access to effective pharmaceuticals while at the same time helping to keep prescription drugs affordable. Health plans should involve participating physicians in developing and reviewing formularies, which should be based on current medical evidence and relevant pharmacoeconomic information and should be regularly reviewed and updated, if necessary on an expedited basis, to take into account new medical evidence and newly approved drugs. In addition, selective formularies should include an exceptions process, directed by a clinician with appropriate expertise, through which a patient or participating physician may present science-based medical evidence to support coverage for a prescription drug not routinely included in the formulary.

Glossary

ABMS (American Board of Medical Specialties)
The oversight and coordinating body for the 24 medical specialty boards.

Accreditation
A process whereby a health care organization (for example, an HMO or hospital) is evaluated by professional reviewers on the basis of a set of predetermined standards.

Board Certified
A doctor who is board certified has been trained in a specialized area of medicine and then passed an exam given by the appropriate medical board approved by the ABMS (e.g., Radiology, Dermatology). Board certification means that the doctor is qualified to practice that specialty.

Board Eligible
Describes a doctor who is eligible to take the exams administered by the approved medical specialty boards. A doctor becomes eligible following graduation from medical school and completion of an approved residency in one of the 25 medical specialties.

Capitation
A method of paying physicians or other providers a set amount of money for the care of patients, rather than paying for each procedure performed.

Case Management

A quality and utilization management technique usually used for patients with complex cases and who may need expensive care.

Cherry Picking

Selecting only the healthiest persons, who are least at risk for illness or injury.

Co-Insurance

Arrangement by which the insurer and the insured share, in a specific ratio, payment for losses covered by the policy, after the deductible is met.

Copayment

The amount paid by a patient for care by a hospital, doctor, or other provider when an insurer pays the remaining portion.

Cost Contracts

Contracts where Medicare pays the HMO a fee to provide hospital and medical services. At the end of the year, if the plan has spent more than Medicare has paid, Medicare reimburses the HMO. Members under this arrangement are able to seek medical services outside the network but are responsible for copayments, deductibles, and extra doctor's charges.

Deductible

The amount paid by the patient for medical care before the insurance company begins to pay. Usually a deductible is calculated on an annual basis; for example, $500 per individual or $1000 per family.

Demand Management

Programs such as nurse information lines, developed to reduce the amount of unnecessary emergency room and/or doctor visits.

Disease State Management

Special programs of prevention and treatment that are established to care for patients with chronic diseases, such as diabetes or hypertension.

Exclusions

A term that refers to the type of benefits or coverages a managed care plan will not cover or reimburse (for example, cosmetic surgery).

Exclusive Provider Organization (EPO)

A group of hospitals, physicians and other providers who provide health care services to covered patients. Patients are covered only within the EPO; if they seek care outside of the network, they must pay for it themselves. *See Preferred Provider Organization.*

Federally Qualified

HMOs that have been evaluated by the Health Care Financing Administration (HCFA) and have met certain standards of quality.

Fee-for-Service

Physician compensation based on services performed. For example, a surgeon receives a specified payment for removing an appendix; a pediatrician receives a specified payment for an office exam.

Formulary

A list of drugs HMOs and hospitals recommend to their doctors for use. A restricted formulary is one where physicians may prescribe only those drugs listed.

Gag Clauses

A clause in an HMO's contract with a doctor that prevents him or her from discussing alternative treatment options with patients.

Gatekeeper

The professional in an HMO who decides whether or not a patient will be referred to a specialist for further care. Physicians, nurses, and physician assistants may all function as gatekeepers.

Group Model HMO

An HMO where the doctors work at a central site. *See Independent Practice Association, Network Model HMO, Staff Model HMO.*

Health Care Financing Administration (HCFA)
Federal agency responsible for Medicare funding. It has a major influence on health policy and finance.

Health Maintenance Organization (HMO)
A managed care organization that combines the functions of a health insurance company and a health care provider.

Indemnity Insurance
A type of insurance where patients pay their bill and then seek reimbursement from the insurance company. There are no restrictions on which doctors or treatments the patient chooses, except for the amount of insurance he or she has. Most indemnity plans reimburse only a portion (80-90 percent) of charges.

Independent Practice Association (IPA)
An HMO where doctors care for patients in their own offices, rather than a central location. *See Group Model HMO, Network Model HMO, Staff Model HMO.*

Managed Care
The integration of health care and health insurance. Managed care is an attempt to control costs and improve quality by using a selected group of providers and, through policy and procedure, managing the care a member of the plan receives.

Managed Indemnity
Indemnity insurance plans that adopt many of the medical management tools of managed care.

Medicaid
A federally sponsored, state managed health insurance program for the poor.

Medicare
A medical insurance program operated by the federal government for people over 65 years of age and/or the disabled.

Medical Loss Ratio

The percentage of total revenue that a health plan spends on medical care.

Mixed Model

A term applied when features of two or more managed care models are combined.

National Committee for Quality Assurance (NCQA)

A voluntary accrediting body for managed care organizations.

Network Model HMO

An HMO made up of groups of doctors, who see patients in their own offices, rather than a central location. Like an IPA, but made up of groups of doctors instead of individual doctors. *See Group Model HMO, Independent Practice Association, Staff Model HMO.*

Outcomes

A term applied to the results of health care. Studies designed to track and measure these results are called outcomes studies.

Per Diem

Term that applies when billing is calculated on a daily rate.

Physician Hospital Organization (PHO)

A managed care model formed primarily by hospitals and their medical staffs in order to negotiate with managed care plans; sometimes called a provider service organization (PSO).

Physician Practice Management (PPM)

Refers to companies that purchase physician practices and networks to negotiate with managed care organizations. These companies will also manage administrative functions such as billing.

Point of Service Plan (POS)

A managed care model sometimes called an open-ended HMO, where patients pay an additional fee for care outside the HMO network.

GLOSSARY

Practice Guidelines
Standardized guidelines for the treatment of diseases or conditions.

Pre-Approval/Authorization
A process where a physician is required to receive prior authorization from a health plan to perform a procedure, hospitalize a patient, or refer a patient to another doctor.

Prepayment Plans
Refers to a contractual arrangement in which Medicare pays an HMO to provide medical services only, not hospital services. Members under this plan can go outside the plan, but are responsible for any copayments, deductibles, or extra doctor's charges.

Pre-existing Condition
A physical or mental disability or illness that a person had before applying for insurance. Insurance companies may refuse to pay for treatment related to a pre-existing condition.

Preferred Provider Organization (PPO)
A group of hospitals, physicians and other providers who provide health care services to covered patients Members are permitted to seek care outside the PPO network, but benefits may be reduced or out-of-pocket costs may be higher. *See Exclusive Provider Organization.*

Preventive Care
Health services that are aimed at maintaining good health and preventing illness, such as routine physical exams, immunizations, and certain diagnostic tests like mammograms or Pap smears.

Primary Care Physician
Once called a general practitioner, this is the physician who is the first to care for a patient's medical needs and who knows the patient on an ongoing basis. In an HMO, the primary care physician is the "gatekeeper," controlling access to other physicians and to hospitals.

Risk Contracts

Contracts where Medicare pays an HMO a monthly sum to provide coverage for Medicare beneficiaries who join. The HMO also usually charges these members a monthly premium to cover the cost of Medicare deductibles and copayments. Members under this plan are not allowed to go outside the plan for care.

Set-Asides

An amount of the money an HMO pays to a doctor that is held back unless he or she succeeds in meeting agreed upon budget goals.

Specialist

A physician who practices medical care in a specialized area of medicine. All physicians who are board certified are specialists, including primary care physicians. In managed care, the term specialist is used somewhat differently; specialists are those doctors to whom primary care physicians refer patients.

Staff Model HMO

A model in which physicians are full-time, salaried employees of the HMO. They practice in one or a limited number of locations. *See Group Model HMO, Independent Practice Association, Network Model HMO.*

Usual and Customary

The methods a health plan uses to determine the average rates charged for medical services. A usual charge is the average of all billed charges from the prior year by a given health care provider for a given procedure. A customary charge is the average of member health care providers' billed charges for the prior year.

Utilization Review

The process of reviewing the care delivered to a patient; the goal is to reduce unnecessary care.

Index

About the Publishers

The mission of Castle Connolly Medical Ltd. is to help individuals and families find the best health care. The company was founded in 1992 by John K. Castle and John J. Connolly, Ed.D.

John K. Castle is the Chairman of Castle Connolly Medical Ltd. He has spent much of the last two decades involved with health care institutions and issues. Mr. Castle served as Chairman of the Board of New York Medical College for eleven years, an institution where he has continued on the Board for more than eighteen years.

Mr. Castle has been extensively involved in other health care and voluntary activities as well. He served for five years as a public commissioner on the Joint Commission on Accreditation of Healthcare Organizations (JCAHO), the body which accredits most public and private hospitals throughout the United States. Mr. Castle has also served as a trustee of three different hospitals in the metropolitan New York region and as a director of the United Hospital Fund, as well as a trustee of the Whitehead Institute.

In addition to his health care activities, Mr. Castle has served on many voluntary boards including the Corporation of the Massachusetts Institute of Technology, as well as numerous corporate boards of directors, including the Equitable Life Assurance Society of the United States. He is chairman of a leading merchant bank and has been chief executive of a major investment bank.

Mr. Castle holds a Bachelor of Science degree from MIT; an MBA with High Distinction from the Harvard Business School, where he was a Baker Scholar; and an honorary doctorate from New York Medical College.

John J. Connolly, Ed.D., is the President and CEO of Castle Connolly Medical Ltd. His experience in health care and education is extensive.

Dr. Connolly served as president of New York Medical College, the state's largest private medical college, for more than ten years. Dr. Connolly is a fellow of the New York Academy of Medicine, a member of the New York Academy of Sciences, a director of the New York Business Group on Health, a member of the President's Council of the United Hospital Fund, and a member of the Media Advisory Board of the Scientists' Institute for Public Information. Dr. Connolly has served as a trustee of two hospitals and as Chairman of the Board of one. He is extensively involved in health care and community activities, and serves on a number of voluntary and corporate boards, including the Board of the American Lyme Disease Foundation, which he chairs, the Friends of the National Library of Medicine, and the Lupus Foundation. He has a Bachelor of Science degree from Worcester State College, a Master's degree from the University of Connecticut, and a Doctor of Education degree in College and University Administration from Teacher's College, Columbia University.